Now the world's most beautiful women tell you how they learned to play the beauty game. Here are their secrets, revealed for the first time, for achieving and maintaining the look of loveliness. Everything from special exercises and dieting to cosmetic surgery and the importance of having the *right* kind of lover. Beauty is a matter of vital concern to Luciana Pignatelli, and she has written a gossipy, amusing, useful book about it—a "survival kit" for women past the first blush of youth.

THE BEAUTIFUL PEOPLE'S BEAUTY BOOK

The Beautiful People's Beauty Book

HOW TO ACHIEVE THE LOOK AND MANNER
OF THE WORLD'S MOST ATTRACTIVE WOMEN

by Princess Luciana Pignatelli
as told to Jeanne Molli

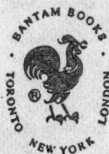

BANTAM BOOKS · TORONTO · LONDON · NEW YORK

A NATIONAL GENERAL COMPANY

*This low-priced Bantam Book
has been completely reset in a type face
designed for easy reading, and was printed
from new plates. It contains the complete
text of the original hard-cover edition.*
NOT ONE WORD HAS BEEN OMITTED.

🚩

THE BEAUTIFUL PEOPLE'S BEAUTY BOOK
*A Bantam Book / published by arrangement with
The McCall Publishing Company*

PRINTING HISTORY
McCall edition published February 1971
2nd printing .... February 1971
3rd printing .... April 1971
4th printing .... May 1971
Cookbook Club edition published August 1971
Extracts appeared in LADIES' HOME JOURNAL *and* VOGUE *in
January 1971,* PAGEANT *in August 1971,* COSMOPOLITAN *in July 1971.*

Bantam edition published May 1972

Cover photograph by Bill King, courtesy of HARPER'S BAZAAR

Published simultaneously in the United States and Canada

PRINTED IN THE UNITED STATES OF AMERICA

Contents

1 How I Learned to Play the Beauty Game

A few times every century, a great natural beauty is born. I an not one of them. But what nature skipped, I supplied—so much so that sometimes I cannot remember what is real and what is fake. More important, neither can anyone else.

When you care about beauty, it may be all to the good if nature is not overgenerous. There is no chance then of living in a mythical past or in perpetual illusion. It does not matter what you start with, try and get by on nature alone past thirty and you are finished. I feel no nostalgia—in fact, I cringe—when I see pictures of myself taken ten years ago. I look better now, at thirty-five, than at any other time in my life. I certainly do not expect an early dotage, nor should anyone nowadays.

One of the international beauties I most admire was a perfect monster at twenty. She did not know how to move or dress. Her hair was thin and her eyes too small. She had bad skin and worse legs. With sheer determination, by thirty she became a subject of envy, by forty a beauty, and the way she is going, she should still be terriffic at eighty. Small wonder that I believe in the long view—in the beauty that survives.

I am a Capricorn, and like most people born under that sign, a late starter. But Capricorn or not, it seems that I had a good beginning. I was a pretty child and very blond, the pride of my German nanny. I also had the advantage of being the youngest and the only girl in a family of three children. My father, Francesco Malgeri, was editor-in-chief of the Rome daily newspaper *Il Messaggero*, until he quarreled with the Fascists. My mother, Nelida Lenci, widow of Count Dino Crespi, had two children by the count, Rudi and Marco Fabio. My early years were spent, together with my parents and half brothers, in an old Roman apartment.

In the summer, my parents would send me to the Crespis' country house in Tuscany, an eleventh-century house with battlements and turrets to climb. The peasant children there were my play-mates. I was very envious of them; they ran around without shoes. Once, when the wheat was cut, I too played barefoot on the stubble—the pain was unbelievable. Thus, my first beauty ambition took form: I would acquire a tough peasant foot. The only part of me that developed fast *was* my feet. They did not look peasant, but were as big at age ten as they are now (size 9½). It was very humiliating; I had to wear men's shoes.

At the war's end, we moved to Brazil. For five years we lived in an old Portuguese colonial house, white, with a tiled roof, beamed ceilings, a patio, and a big garden. I loved the house but hated myself. I was becoming a monster. My wisdom teeth came through early and all wrong. By the time they were pulled, they had made my front teeth buck out. To correct this, I was forced to stand in front of the mirror saying "p" over and over again to bring the upper lip down. Meanwhile, my nose grew thick and so did my waist. I was also made to wear a girdle—a terrible mistake for a young girl, though common practice at the time. A girdle does the work that muscles should be taught to do. Wear one for a number of years and the result is a flabby behind.

I was a lump, and everyone knew it. To compound the dreariness, my parents sent me to a school run by nuns. All legs and big feet, thick at the waist and thick in the nose, with no breasts and droopy shoulders, I had only one dream—I would grow up to be madly sexy like the movie stars of the forties with their curves and cleavage. I longed for big breasts. In Brazil, where girls mature early, all my friends already had bosoms. I had only a chest. The sole favorable omen was Aunt Dora, who was remarkably endowed. I hoped this meant that bosoms ran in the family, not that anyone ever mentioned them—they were always referred to obliquely as "Dora's hearts."

Later, I began to try on another image, the svelte woman. In view of my thick, if shapeless, proportions, this was just as farfetched as sexy curves but, with great diligence, I began to collect pictures of beautiful, chic, slender ladies from fashion magazines. Most unhappy adolescents do moon over them. They know that such women must be models of loveliness or their pictures would not be published.

It was during my svelte stage that my brother Rudi arrived in Brazil with his wife, Consuelo, née O'Connor. She and her twin sister, Gloria, had been the most photographed debutantes of their year and became top New York models. Even in real life, Consuelo had that magazine glamour. One morning I was asked to awaken Consuelo. She had always seemed too beautiful to be true, and this was my chance to find out. She was asleep, but up close I could see that even asleep with no makeup, she looked great.

Later that morning, Consuelo let me try on some of her clothes. I struggled into them, and they almost fit. Rudi had brought me a bikini from America that I also modeled. The bikini fit me, but the shape it revealed was pathetic. Thinking, I suppose, that at least something could be done about my droopy shoulders, Rudi suggested that they might be the problem. He and Consuleo showed me a basic shoulder exercise. For months, whenever I had a spare moment alone, I would raise my arms to shoulder height, swing them to the front, cross them twice quickly, hold for two counts, thrust arms to the sides, hold two counts, back to the front, cross quickly, back to the sides. . . . One, two, three, four; one, two, three, four. The shoulders began to respond. Had I sprouted wings, I could not have been more proud.

Later, when I came to Rome to visit the Crespis, I tried on some of Consuelo's clothes again. It was a moment of triumph for me. I probably looked ridiculous, as most young girls do in clothes that are too old for them, but I thought I looked divine. They bought me a pretty, fashionable dress that was right for me. Clothes do "make the man"—I improved instantly.

Rudi also suggested some lipstick. My little bit of lipstick went unnoticed and was subsequently allowed (I was fifteen). But my progress was stopped when I bought some dark stockings, rather daring for the period. The first time he saw me in them, Marco Fabio protested, in front of my parents, that I looked like a streetwalker. The stockings had to go.

I was shipped off to a girls' school at Brillantmont in Lausanne. I missed the Brazilian sun, the white and purple flowers, the *azulejo* tiles. In a word, I hated boarding school where everyone had to be one of the group. My savings went for stamps, chocolate, and beauty products. My greatest discovery at the local drugstore was an eyelash curler, the kind you clamp on and then twist—the sort that millions of women still struggled with in the fifties. I thought that using the curler and a little bit of dark vaseline made a great difference.

I confided these beauty experiments to an aunt who lived in Rome. My parents, on a visit to her house, read one of my letters. It was the letter in which I told all!—how I practiced with the curler and how adept I had become. My parents took it as a family tragedy, a scandal to be smothered. It was the equivalent then of discovering today that your daughter smokes pot. But when I came to Rome with my lashes curled, my mother thought I looked very good.

By this time I spoke French, English, and Portuguese as well as Italian (my early German had been forgotten except for the nursery words one never forgets). It gave me a semblance of confidence to realize I was no longer the provincial I had been. I was allowed to finish school in Rome on one condition. My father, who had started the weekly magazine *Settimana Incom,* insisted I work for him after school. At seventeen, I hated work. I was the most frivolous thing on earth. All I really wanted to do, aside from becoming beautiful, was to ride horses, which I did every day. I liked horses so much my parents worried about it.

They did not know that there was more to worry about than my excessive infatuation with horses. The fresh air and exercise had slimmed me down, and I had grown slightly prettier. In Italy, you are instantly aware of the effect this has on men. A playboy with a mustache, who thought I was rich, had started to flirt with me on the bridle path. He was probably a very obvious Latin-lover stereotype, but when he came riding, with his white turtleneck sweater setting off an impeccable tan, to me he was the most beautiful man on earth. If this marvel of marvels was interested in me, maybe I was not as hopeless as I had feared. The idea was so encouraging that I stole off to a beauty salon for my first facial and massage. I could not go openly; it was not done at the time.

I still believed that big breasts were indispensable and it bothered me that mine were anything but big. (Now I confess it is a relief not to have to worry about their upkeep.) The sympathetic owner of the salon gave me an infrared treatment and a massage. She also suggested that, to help the bosom along, I drink a lot of beer. I detested beer, but I drank it. Instead of getting big breasts, I began to get a rather big behind.

The romance at the riding ring faded, and with that my mania for horses was lost in the shuffle of new events. When I turned eighteen, Rudi gave me a coming-out party. I was written up as one of the young beauties of Rome. I was willing to grant that I had improved, but not that much. I knew I was very unphotogenic, which left me in terror of photographers. Henry Clarke did the one picture of me with my old nose in which I looked well. I think I have destroyed all other pictures of me at this age.

Only through Rudi could I convince my parents to let me have my nose done. Mother always agreed with his suggestions. With him as my ally, my parents consented. We decided on England, because that was the best place for cosmetic surgery at the time. When my mother and I entered Sir Archibald McIndoe's office, he asked, with perfect tact, which of us wanted her nose redone. (There was nothing wrong with Mother's.) He worked out three designs for me. I immediately chose the one that was a cross between Vivien Leigh's and Consuelo's. As the operation neared, all I could do was keep praying, "My God, I hope I chose well."

The anesthesia may have been a bit strong. I slept for twelve hours and came out of it totally bewildered, with a form of amnesia. I did not know where I was, only that I wanted to go home. My mother shrieked, "They redid her nose and touched her brain," but five days later I was sightseeing all over London with my nose in a plaster. The explanations were that I had had an automobile accident or fallen in the bathroom. After three weeks, we left London.

According to the doctor's prognosis, it would take almost a year for the new nose to take its final shape. When I first got back to Rome, Rudi saw my swollen face and said, "It's not possible, she's worse than before." But seawater and sun work miracles. After one month with relatives in Calabria, the nose was set and mine.

It was such a wonderful feeling that whether the

effect was more psychological than real is incidental. I felt much surer of myself than before. Still, for added confidence whenever there was an invitation to a cocktail party, I went over to Rudi's first so that we could enter together.

Marshall McLuhan, in his usual provocative manner, once said: "Cosmetic and clothing advertisers assume everybody wants to be beautiful. Actually, lots of people want to be ugly. It is safer. Being beautiful forces one out into life; so they put life away by cultivating ugliness. This is not done consciously, of course, but it is nonetheless a major effort by a lot of frightened people."

Perhaps. I know that with my old nose I had hated public exposure because I did not feel equipped to handle it. I was frightened because in Rome I was surrounded by glamorous, sophisticated, beautiful people—or so they seemed to me—and I did not measure up. But everyone is forced out into life. I could not imagine anyone wanting to be ugly. Now I see lots of these ostriches, some of them lazy, some of them not, who seem to feel their beauty is immune. They do all the wrong things as if tomorrow will never come. I do not know whether or not this is a major self-destructive effort. But what I notice even more is people who could be far more attractive if they only met someone who could show them how. Sparking beauty is like sparking the mind. If you are lucky, early in your life a wise person says something to you that strikes home, something that points you in the right direction, and you carry on from there. I was lucky, I had Rudi. His grand manner, good taste, and good advice always proved invaluable to me.

Six months after my nose surgery, I married Prince Nicolò Pignatelli Aragona Cortes. I was the envy of Rome for this brilliant match. My husband was one of the most charming men one can think of, but he had almost too many qualities, and the marriage was a disaster. I looked like hell in a photograph Dick Avedon took of me early in the marriage. I used to have facials constantly that never did any good. And yet, without them, I might have looked worse.

I was in crisis and heeded the old folklore that babies save a marriage. My daughter, Fabrizia, was born in 1956, followed by my son, Diego, in 1958. Everyone says how divine it is to have a beautiful baby and how lucky one is to have a nanny to help. The first one was all terribly British and chic, the kind that thinks anyone born south of Calais is a savage. She arrived from London and quit before the baby was born. We had seven nannies the first year. The first months were terrible; there was something wrong with the baby's formula, and my daughter almost died when her weight at four months dropped to her weight at birth. I finally found a wet nurse for her—you still could fourteen years ago.

After the baby, I was so afraid of losing my figure that I became too thin. Rather than taking it easy, I rushed straight back into Roman life with the result that I was tired and sick for a year. My doctor told me not to worry, all I really needed was a lover. This idea shocked me.

When my son was born, I had the good sense to rest. We went to the shore, where I was a "milking cow" on the beach, soaking up sun and swimming between feedings. Still it was no good.

Nursing is supposed to benefit the child and compels the mother to lead a well-regulated life. It did wonders for both my looks and health, but for the baby's sake never nurse when you are quarreling with your husband all the time. In my case, it did not stop the flow, but all the arguments came out in the milk. The baby screamed eighteen hours a day.

My *idée fixe* during and after pregnancy was that I was stuck forever with the wrong man. We lived in an old house with bad tempers, screaming children, and leaking roofs. Marriage takes so much organization and stuffs the two of you so close together you can see love dying all over the walls.

One of the problems about the marriage, doubtless, was my feeling of not knowing how to cope with our social life and entertaining. Dolce vita or no dolce vita, my husband's attitude remained traditionalist, and this called for formal dinner parties of stifling tedium. For my first party, the tablecloth had to be brocade; the silver English; the roses red, and the menus engraved in gold.

Hours were spent in organizing, and I must have checked the table setting five times before the guests arrived. Despite this, instead of a gold-engraved menu, one guest's was blank. My husband's secretary had been enlisted to send out the invitations so there could be no mistakes, but a man quite clearly invited alone brought his wife, which threw off the protocol of the seating arrangement.

I thought at the time that a butler had to be seven feet tall and dressed in livery with the family crest and colors. After my interviews, I was sure I had found exactly the man I needed. Just before the party, my dream butler, while trying to start a blaze in the fireplace, managed to destroy the flue with a poker. Smoke invaded the room like killer smog.

One evening, just as I was beginning to gain confidence with these grim soirées, I discovered upon entering the dining room that it was raining on the centerpiece through a leak in the roof. Now, I would simply move the table, put up an umbrella and relax, but inexperienced, at twenty-one, I was shattered.

I believe in lucky and unlucky houses and in happy and unhappy cycles. In my ex-husband's house, everyone was unhappy, even the parrot. It was my fault, too. With two strong personalities, either you pull together or you destroy each other. What does this have to do with beauty? Lots! No one who has ever seen or felt it questions the glow that happiness gives. For helping your looks, the emotional security and teamwork of a good marriage is unbeatable. The trick I had to learn early was to keep going no matter what. This takes a strong dose of ego—or just plain selfishness. If loving care is so good for people, one might as well lavish some on oneself.

If anyone understands this, it is the model-actress Veruschka, one of the most glamorous Romans-by-adoption. Veruschka (Countess Vera von Lehndorff) was born in Königsberg (now Kaliningrad) on the Gulf of Danzig. Her officer father was shot during the war because of his participation in the anti-Hitler plot of July, 1944. She spent her youth wandering through West Germany with her mother and three sisters. They would stay wherever friends had room and food and could take them in.

In this migrant life, Veruschka changed schools fifteen times. The first one to have meaning for her was an art school in Hamburg. This prompted her to scrimp for a trip to Florence to do watercolors of

Renaissance glories. A local photographer decided it was Veruschka who was glorious and asked her to do some fashion modeling. The rest is magazine-cover history.

"If you never sleep, or smoke like crazy, or never go out in the air," Veruschka says, "it shows. But if you're not happy, that's what shows the most. Some evenings, I can spend two hours in front of the mirror and nothing fantastic happens. I'm depressed and convinced it can't, but I try. Other evenings, I put a little black here and there—put a little black on my spirit—and I look great."

In other words, what do you do when you are depressed? Look terrible for the duration? I think not. You do what Veruschka does on an off evening. You struggle with the mirror anyhow. The evening might improve.

During my marriage, I realized that frustration was making me ugly. My instinct was to preserve my looks as much as possible. Even if the immediate results were not exactly knockout, I figured I might be happier later. But if I lost my looks, that prospect would be dimmed.

Mind you, it works both ways. Observing other people, I now realize that happiness does not in itself guarantee that you will look marvelous—not unless you use that happy glow only as a starting point and then really work at it. The three-way mirror in the bathroom cannot kindle that little old light in the eyes, but it can be a shattering reflection when all one has to show is inner radiance.

One of the more devastating adopted Romans, Gore Vidal, gives a verdict on beauty that indeed destroys the comforting platitudes: "Beauty is exterior; it is not interior," he says. "Not only does it not matter if there's nothing inside, it probably helps. Character has a tendency to ruin looks. Will, however, can reconstruct a face pretty much to order. Read Hegel. Read Anita Colby."

Before, during, or after marriage, happy or unhappy, I underwent hypnosis, had cell implants, diacutaneous fibrolysis, silicone injections, my nose bobbed, and my eyelids lifted. I have tried aromatotherapy, approached yoga, and still go to the best gymnast in Rome. Facials and pedicures are normal routine, as are frequent hair and makeup changes. I will try anything new in beauty. I could not bear not to try. I must have experimented with every gadget on the market—and discarded most. (We'll talk about specifics later.) Still, the idea is to leave some time for enjoying what beauty helps to bring.

Talitha Getty* is a girl who enjoys life but also takes good care of herself. A swinging, chestnut-blond beauty, fey and fine-boned, she is a health food addict, as is her husband, Paul Getty, Jr. She is also mad for massage. Talitha was born Dutch and raised in the exuberant Augustus John family circle in England. Home is now Rome, London, and Marrakesh. She adores the exotic and romantic, the silken East and caftaned Africa. She travels there on her husband's business trips. Talitha's outlook on beauty is at once simple and aware: "Even the most hideous people look beautiful when they're in love. With a good man, a woman doesn't need treatments, health foods, vitamins, or anything . . . not at first."

I might add that finding the wrong man is disaster. For example, the man attracted by your glamour who then proceeds to tell you that you would be much lovelier with your hair down and your eyes unmade; the man who cannot see why a few pounds

* Since publication, Talitha Getty died tragically, July 14, 1971.

(which sink straight to the rear) could possibly do any harm. It is such a boring attitude, and when heeded, leads always to the same boring result. You take away this, take away that, and in six months you look like a cook.

By the end of one affair, I had really become very plain-looking—almost nothing on my face, nothing on my nails, the most casual clothes. I saw the man two years later and he told me, "I didn't realize you were so beautiful." I no longer was when we broke up. But when we first met I certainly had not been plain or he would not have looked at me. Heaven only knows why so many real men have this destructive approach—men who apparently are neither overpossessive nor jealous. I suppose they want you to look natural because they equate it with bed.

While on the subject of men, a brief, loud hurrah for homosexuals and their incredible eye for line, proportion, detail, and style. As a Rome magazine writer said: "Every woman over thirty needs a homosexual in her life." She needs someone who is genuinely interested in making her look better, perhaps because it is his business. Homosexuals, particularly those in the beauty and fashion field, are both expert and generous with their knowledge. Husbands and lovers cannot be bothered or, if they do spot defects, cannot tell you how to correct them. It is not the reason you are with them. I even believe in separate bedrooms—much more conducive to sex—so I am not about to point out the latest wrinkle, emotional or otherwise, to the man in my life, at least not until I can deal with it myself.

Men are here to stay and they are great. If you want to keep your looks, hold on to the good men by all means, but get rid of the ones who put you down. Some women need very little love, and others base their whole life on it. A woman consumed by a bad affair may destroy herself entirely or have far more trouble keeping an inner balance than the one who does not need love at any price. Regarding men, take it from a knowledgeable woman who never figured as a bluestocking in anybody's book: "You're never too old to become younger," said Mae West in a *Look* interview. "I'm just happy with myself. If I find a man absorbs too much of my time and my mind, and makes me concentrate on him, I get rid of him. It's all right for a man to concentrate on me. Keep doing things you like to do. Have people around you who think and feel the same way as you do—who needs 'no' men around?"

After my husband and I separated, Brazil was my good thing. The place was right, the man there was right—Mae West was right. I needed a change of scene, and the warm, free-and-easy social life of Rio was the perfect solution. Whatever unconventionality I possess, I owe in large measure to Brazil. It was there I began to enjoy life, instead of forcing it into a mold. I began to realize that marriage and position, protocol and propriety are not all that important. They pale when you go swimming on the beaches at Angra dos Reis where orchids grow down to the sea.

I edged back into Europe via Portugal, hoping that outpost might be a way of keeping both worlds. I kept neither and spent a year doing nothing at all. I was so bored I used to remove the hairs from my legs, one by one, with tweezers. It was time to come home.

I took a small ground-floor apartment in Palazzo Taverna. If it was to be Rome, it would be old Rome—a splashing fountain in a cobblestoned courtyard, a carved wooden front door, vaulted ceilings, gilt and red-velvet furnishings. But it would not be all Roman. From South America I brought a collection of irregularly cut amethysts that I kept loose in a silver bowl and from Portugal, a church carving and a rug woven by women in jail for murder.

When I first came back, I still needed traditional reassurance. But I had learned a lot. First of all, turning thirty is not like taking the veil. In my case, it was more like crossing the Rubicon. I had two young children and I was on my own. In the conventional Italian view, at that time, a woman in this situation, even with money, was supposed to be frustrated and desperate. Presumably she would sit by the telephone and cry. I, on the contrary, had never had more friends and men around me in my life. The men were not Italian, though; having once married the ultimate in Italian men, and having found him insupportable, why persist? Romance involved plane tickets, but no one stays put in one place anymore. Men adore to catch planes, and so do I. No one objects to cruising around the Mediterranean either.

I was lucky to find Miss Huzy Kano, the best nanny in the world, for my children. She is still with me. My daughter now goes to La Combe, a Swiss boarding school, and writes me about her beauty as well as her scholastic progress. Fabrizia is no false sophisticate—I detest that in young girls —but I do encourage her to keep her teenage hair, skin, and figure in the best possible condition so that mistakes will not have to be undone later. My son lives with me in Rome and goes to public school.

Once settled, I looked for something to do. I did boutique clothes, only to discover that you have to be a lot tougher than I am to run that sort of production. The designer would see everything in red and black for a season. If the customer did not like clothes in combinations of red and black, she could drop dead as far as he was concerned. He was interested in presenting a collection that would make good copy for the press. It did not matter to him whether or not the collection sold. In addition, the seamstresses, typically Italian, with all their personal and family problems, would find new excuses to show up later and later every morning.

Eventually, I changed both my business and my surroundings. I needed more space, and the idea of twentieth-century convenience and high-rise sunshine more than compensated for the loss of Palazzo Taverna's old-world charm. Installed in a modern apartment, I began to look inward to find what I should do. Friends had always turned to me for advice, and I realized that beauty counseling came naturally to me. It was about time I put all the lessons I had learned into practice. Beauty, once a hobby and always an obsession, became my vocation. I have been doing fashion coordination and product development work for almost two years now. This entails frequent trips to the United States and England. It means I always have to look my best, but that is what I like to do.

When you become involved deeply in any discipline—and beauty, above all, is discipline—it takes you outside of yourself. First, you learn to see your own looks as a quality apart from self, as a symbol, "a thing." This leads in turn to an immediate appraisal of other beauties and an understanding of the whole problem and phenomenon. In reaching out, you see that all women can be in the game together, and you find that you want to help the others play.

2 Discipline, Dawn to Dawn

I believe in dazzle and in learning all the tricks and flourishes that can make a woman glamorous. Still, one has to learn to take things in sequence—glamour can begin only when all the groundwork has been laid. Your looks depend on your discipline. In beauty terms, discipline means controlling the way you eat, the hours you sleep, and the amount of exercise you take. In the broadest sense, discipline encompasses the balance you strike between work and relaxation. Makeup, hairstyle, and chic can add the dazzle that makes you a striking beauty, but their effects are transient unless they are sustained by stringent living habits.

Before designing your own beauty routine, you have to evaluate your life-style in terms of its effect on your appearance. The work you do, the man or men in your life, and the number of children you have all play a part in determining the amount of time you have to spend on yourself. By time for yourself I mean not only time spent with beauty preparations, but time relaxing and enjoying life as well. Too many of us run ourselves ragged trying to be mistress, wife, mother, perfect housekeeper, hostess, and career woman all at once. This is nonsense but often happens unless we are sure of what we want.

If it seems that you have no time at all, you might try listing what you do with your time, hour by hour, for a week. Surely one afternoon or evening a week can be set aside for beauty. I would rather be complimented on my looks than on my cakes, which is not to say that baking is bad for you, but only that something has to be sacrificed and it need not be your looks. If anyone objects, candidly announce that this is your selfish day.

Remember, too, that locale is important. Environment always interacts with your looks, no matter what your beauty type. Making the surroundings function in your favor is a universal problem. Sometimes I envy the smooth, relaxed faces of friends who live in the suburbs or in the country. It is tempting to think that anyone would look as marvelous in those pleasant surroundings, but fresh air and quiet alone do not give them their serene appearance; it is adoring the country life and knowing how to live it that works wonders. As with so many other things, it matters less what you begin with than what you do with what you have.

I adore city life. Living in the city, though, one finds that it requires more effort to maintain self-discipline. The sedentary, noisy, high-tension atmosphere of most cities hardly fosters a radiant glow. One must learn to moderate all of the diversions and entertainments that make city life attractive, or they will take their toll in beauty. Of all cities, Rome is my first love, but it is a tricky town to cope with, one requiring highly disciplined habits. This is because Rome's pace, charm, and geography equally favor personal beauty and the *laisser-aller* attitude that destroys it.

On the one hand, beautiful women in Rome take full advantage of living in one of the last of the pleasurable big cities. They enjoy the food and wine; they enjoy the sky and sun; they are waited on and rarely rushed. Romans have time for each other as well as for work. They have time to sit in the sun in the winter, and when summer comes, time to escape behind drawn shutters. They look out over flowered terraces, move through piazzas and rooms of excellent proportions. Friends call up at the last minute: "Let's go out to lunch . . . dinner . . . the country . . . the shore." Other friends arrive from abroad. If they are celebrities, they are made much of, but so are most visitors to Rome. No matter who the client, waiters hover discreetly in restaurants, way past closing time.

Nothing ever functions as it should; but, for one reason or another, nothing ever does in any big city. At least the Romans, who have never made efficiency a point of honor, take the deficiencies in stride. In their fashion, they work as hard and as long as anyone else—they merely string their workday out with a long break in the middle instead of packing it tight. The long break gives us two fresh starts to the day. We have time to nap or to drive to a pool and back in the summer.

On the other hand, in Rome many more people seem to be working on different wavelengths and schedules than in other urban centers, and many of the women are not working at all. One has to create one's own work hours and one's own discipline and beauty routine, or the years go by, one is never alone, nothing is accomplished, and fat has invaded body and brain.

Romans are still deliciously old-fashioned enough to like or dislike you for what you are—for *simpatia*. They do not worship the cult of success, and as far as beauty is concerned, an early transition from young delectables into mamas and matrons is taken as a matter of course.

There are few pressures in Rome, and without outside pressure, the onus of developing discipline is placed squarely on the individual. At bottom, that is where it always is, but in Rome perhaps more than elsewhere. There is nothing hateful about the surroundings to fight against or to escape from through work, nothing compulsive in the mentality about staying in shape. You alone have to wish to make something of yourself.

"Everyone complains they are a bit tired," says Consuelo Crespi. Consuelo is American, not Italian, but she has lived in Rome so many years she has absorbed the style by osmosis. Her Romanization has reached the point where she and her New York-based sister, Gloria, look like the only twins in the world who could have been born in different countries. "Blame the fatigue on the sirocco," Consuelo says. "Yet life is more casual, less demanding in Rome. The mood is good. In New York, you instantly sense the heavy pressure and responsibility. Here pressures creep up more insidiously, but we have them, and at some point they have to be faced intelligently—you start cutting down."

The first things one gives up, of course, are those that are least painful. For example, Consuelo admits, "Nightclubs don't amuse me, and I never go except if under an obligation. Thank God, that's over with."

I have always been convinced that work is not bad for your looks, but agree that staying out all night in stuffy nightclubs is, and it only steals time better spent in bed asleep, alone or otherwise. Early-evening cocktail parties—those standing bores—

are rare in Rome, replaced by the more civilized dinner invitation. This eliminates the agony of toying with a glass of tonic water for two hours rather than loading up on liquor that your face and body cannot take. I am no Carrie Nation, but getting drunk for dinner is just plain stupid.

Consuelo, who is Italian editor for *Vogue*, has her own system for deadline pressures and twelve-hour working days covering fashion collections. Once home, she refuses anything but a hot bath and total relaxation.

"I see no one when work is over for the day. I pretend I'm out of town," she says. "No makeup, no hairdo, no effort. The evening is total quiet and early to bed."

Consuelo exaggerates, of course. Not even in darkest Africa would she relax without her hair done and face made up, but she does know how to change pace and totally relax, one of the most important beauty tricks to learn. Even on a normal, more leisurely schedule, her routine is to find a half hour of oblivion before dressing for the evening. She puts on a bossa nova or Burt Bacharach record, stretches out, and in twenty minutes can recoup and reorganize life. She calls it "pulling out the plug." Another of Consuelo's habits, except in summer, is to replace the long lunchbreak siesta with a drive up to Villa Borghese for a walk in the park.

"I believe in organization, and in working," Consuelo says. "Working gives you a sense of accomplishment and lends perspective to the day. If I hadn't worked, I would have been completely hysterical raising children. [She has two, Brando, twenty-one, and Pilar, nineteen.] Instead, the energies are distributed, and when one can relax, one enjoys it so much more."

My own routine now is to work half days in Rome and around the clock on business trips. When home, my basic discipline is to eat and drink little, smoke less, and walk miles. Recently, I switched from five cigarettes a day to five long, narrow Filipino cigars. They have more flavor, and I defy you to smoke more than five a day.

Having a dog, as I do, usually helps you to get out and walk, bcause you feel it is immoral to keep the animal cooped up all the time. My dog, José Bonifacio, unfortunately is one of the laziest, if most lovable, basset hounds in the world. He prefers bed to the outdoors. If I counted on his promptings, I would not walk an inch. During business trips when I am closed in for hours in hotel rooms with meetings and interviews, I try to get some air by hiking around the block—much better than a coffee break. In Rome, I also arrange to exercise regularly at the gym, have pedicures, and see the trichologist about the health of my hair. These are habits that I consider basic to health and beauty for sedentary city life.

Discipline also means always finding time to be impeccable for an appointment. Looking like a frump in public simply is not acceptable—not even to pick up toothpaste at the drugstore. Perhaps this attitude is natural to me because of my parents' example. Both of them make the effort to stay in top form at all times. My mother's beauty plan is simple. As she says, "I don't smoke, I don't drink, and I go to bed early. I exercise and I walk two and a half miles every day." After she turned sixty, she also had her face lifted.

Despite all my careful plans, my parents' example, and my sense of beauty discipline, there is one big snag—I suffer from insomnia. Every one I know sleeps beautifully in Rome, so it must be me, not the environment. I have heard dozens of theories on the causes of insomnia: fear of death, being so geared up one cannot stop, or a perfectionism that makes one rehash the day and plan ahead for the next instead of sleeping. Whatever the cause, the seizures are exhausting. I tried hypnosis in New York, where it is a more commonplace cure than in Rome. It helped, but I never stay there long enough to follow up.

When I am on a tight schedule and cannot compensate with afternoon naps, I take sleeping pills. They work, but I refuse to make them a habit.

Getting to bed by midnight tames the monster more than anything else for me. And someday, when I have more time, I shall go back to yoga. When I practiced it, I started to yawn in the middle of the day and lost all sense of time. Perhaps had I stayed with it longer, I would have hit upon the proper rhythm.

My yogi, Grant Muradoff, Russia's loss and Rome's gain, was pleased I felt like yawning. He believes that, far from being a sign of boredom, yawning charges the batteries and gives you strength. It is one of the simplest rejuvenators anyone can find.

I hope you are never plagued by insomnia, but if you are, you know it takes various forms. I, for example, have no trouble falling asleep; I drop off instantly. My difficulty lies in not being able to stay asleep a sufficient number of hours. It is with this type of insomnia that my experience may be helpful. First of all, I was pleased to see that Mura-doff confirms my intuition that going to bed later does not make you sleep longer. He cites the advice that Prince Felix Youssoupov, the man who killed Rasputin, was given by his father. The young prince was told always to be in bed before midnight. If he wanted to get up at two or three o'clock to go out and dance, that was all right, as long as he did not miss his early sleep. The prince was also enjoined, no matter what time he got back to bed on the nights he left it, always to observe his regular morning rising time, shave, and have breakfast. Then, if he wished, he could go back to bed. The regular sleep-inducing pattern was preserved.

I, like most of my contemporaries, not only have to get up early, I have to stay up. In Rome, I can take a nap in the afternoon; I can't when I am traveling. The yogi approach to insomnia makes sense. In our terms, it roughly translates: If you can't beat them, join them. When Muradoff cannot sleep, rather than fret about early morning obligations, he switches on the light, gets out his yarrow sticks, and practices *I Ching*, from the Chinese book of wisdom and prophecy. I write a letter or read a book. I know I will probably feel exhausted later in the day, but worrying about it will only make me look worse. I do the yoga "elephant swing," I get up, take a standing position with feet apart and arms hanging loose, sway to the left, sway to the right, and so on. It puts me either back to sleep or in such a frame of mind that staying awake is tolerable.

Beauty discipline, in the case of insomnia, means learning to live with a problem until it works itself out. My insomnia usually strikes when I am working or traveling under pressure. It also attacks, I now realize, whenever I feel that all the responsibility is squarely on my shoulders. When I am cruising on a yacht, there is no problem. When there is someone around who cares, it gives me such emotional security I could sleep until noon.

Former cover girl Mirella Petteni Haggiag is a beauty who is as active as I am and who feels the same compulsion to be superorganized and hyper-perfectionist. Yet for her sleep is no stumbling block. She could easily sleep more; she makes herself get up. Mirella rarely gets to bed before 2 A.M. and still shines at 7:30 A.M. I am opposed to getting to bed so late. She seems to thrive, but then she usually naps an hour or so in the afternoon to compensate. When her breakfast tray arrives, she picks up a bed-table agenda and gets herself organized, making lists and phone calls. On vacation, she still wakes up early, has breakfast, and then—shades of Youssoupov—goes back to bed until noon.

"I like to drink in the evening," she says. "Having a bottle of wine with friends is important. I'm the anxious type that programs everything, but I also like good living. When I'm traveling or away on country weekends, I eat anything I want."

The basics of her discipline come from her modeling days. As a model, appointments had to be kept, instant adjustments made and the desired effect produced, no matter how she felt.

Tall, slender, dark-haired, with a superb pre-Renaissance profile, Mirella now has two children and three houses, works for Cole of California in Italy, and is Rome editor for Italian *Vogue*. Meanwhile, she accompanies her husband, movie producer Roberto Haggiag, on business trips three to four months of the year.

"Having been a model—and I was a real professional—I know I'll always retain a certain body knowledge. If I cross my legs at eighty, I'll cross them right. I take care of my looks because it helps give me an inner balance and self-respect. But my life is full. As a model I used to have vast complexes about fanny and hips. Now a pound more or less doesn't matter."

Mirella, who weighted thirty pounds more when she was a teenager, is convinced that weight is a question of nerves and your approach to food. When you think food, you get fat. For lunch in Rome, she cuts carbohydrate intake two or three days a week, eating only meat, eggs, cheese, and fruit. She believes that vegetables make her fat, so she takes vitamin and mineral pills in their place. Working out in a gym several times a week fits into her schedule more easily than sports. Shots of vitamin B12 pick her up when she is overly tired. Once every ten days, she has the works: hair done, a facial and mask, hand, arm, and elbow massage. The idea is that for one afternoon it is important to be the most important person, to indulge, splurge, and be taken care of.

I must say almost any busy woman can arrange one blissfully sybaritic afternoon every week or ten days. If a woman does not, it is time to reconsider the way she organizes life. It might be an evening rather than an afternoon. It might be do-it-yourself rather than having it done for you, but the morale boost of a few hours' total concentration on beauty is enormous. It puts one on keel for days.

To my mind, the most striking example of balance and discipline in Rome is Sophia Loren. It is as if she took her insecurities and, by sheer force of will, turned them inside out and made them work for her. Sophia has always insisted she is shy, and no one ever believes her. But it may be that only a basically shy person would find a way to appear so self-confident.

Sophia's hands are rarely still when she talks, but this is probably due more to being Neapolitan than being nervous. Whatever the cause, the movement of the long fingers that turn up slightly at the tips is a study in controlled elegance. As for Sophia's devastating walk, if that is shy, I am Minnie Mouse.

When Sophia films, it is a twelve-hour day, and her life revolves around it. Between films, she rarely sets foot off the grounds of her villa near Rome. She flies off to an important gala, to Paris for fittings, or dines out in Rome with a visiting VIP, but these are "special events, they aren't life."

Some people cannot take success—they do not know what to do with it. Sophia preferred to stay quietly at home when she was a girl. She prefers it now. Old friends, women she trusts and likes, come out to see her. They listen to records, swim in the pool, and play cards.

Home is six acres and a fifty-room house, classified as an official Italian monument, probably built in the sixteenth century by a prince of the Church. There are catacombs under the main building and a cave out by the guest house. Eighteenth-century ceilings and frescoes have been restored and paneling installed from old churches. The more formal rooms are furnished with brocades, marble-topped tables, enormous mirrors, and statuary. A new wing contains a large modern sitting room, with paintings by Modigliani and Bacon and a Renoir terracotta mother and child. She takes no credit; Carlo Ponti did the whole place, down to the last demitasse cup.

"If you don't have discipline of body and spirit, you can't be an actress," Sophia says, "unless you're a bad one. The only pill I take is vitamin C—I'm afraid of getting the flu. I don't follow any particular regimen at the moment. I never eat in the morning, except for three or four cups of coffee. But that's because I'm Neapolitan. I go to bed at nine. Carlo likes to go to bed early, too. Before, when I smoked, I would stay up later. Now I start yawning."

Sophia is used to getting up early for work and always wakes at seven. Regular hours may sound dull, but they are one of the oldest beauty recipes. Night people often are very charming, yet, in my experience, they almost never keep their looks.

Sophia also used to nap a few hours in the afternoon. Now she spends the time with Carlo, Jr., instead. Almost every Italian woman acts like the "Mother of Italy" when she has her first child. No one teases Sophia about it because she tried so long to have one. To avoid yet another miscarriage when pregnant with Carlo, Jr., she went to Geneva and remained confined to her room for seven months. Having a child has given her deeper confidence as a woman. Becoming a mother does that to almost all of us. It shows in Sophia's face.

Visiting with her at her house, one has the feeling that at last here is someone who knew just what she wanted, and got it. On a movie set, she is a hard-working professional. At home, she now reigns like a queen who has produced the heir apparent.

Virginia Ira von und zu Furstenberg, on the other hand, was born a princess and is learning to be a movie star. Italian on her mother's side, with her dark hair, rounded form, and sensuous mouth, Ira is the picture of luscious self-indulgence. Yet her basic regime is austere. She is early to bed, early to rise, and does not smoke or drink. In Rome, between films and traveling, she goes to a gym every day for two hours.

Ira, who puts on weight easily, knows she has to be disciplined about eating. She says that when you have to watch calories, it is much easier if you eat alone. This does not mean you have to give up men's company, but ideally, you should have a man who is not always around. A man, she says, loves to go out to eat. He orders pasta or curry with rice, and how can one resist? And so often if your man has worked late, you are starving, and dietary prudence goes out the window.

When Ira is alone, she skips lunch or orders just salad and mozzarella cheese. When she does a film, the tension makes her lose weight. But she tries to avoid rapid ups and downs. The trouble when you lose weight quickly from fatigue and tension is that everything falls. Ira's diet pills and diuretics gave her palpitations and she stopped taking them. Her system now is to avoid any reliance on pills. She is afraid that if the body gets too accustomed to pills, it will not work anymore when you stop.

"I used to have an elaborate regimen in Paris," she says. "I went to a gym, to a sauna, to Payot for hand massage, to another place for electric massage, and to Carita for facials. But you have to have nothing else on your mind to keep this up. It was becoming my whole life, and it wasn't worth it."

I understand Ira's food temptations. One would have to be more insensitive than a stone not to be tempted in Italy. Rome is an eat-late-and-linger town. This is particularly the case in good weather, when one can eat outdoors in the country under grape arbors, surrounded by prowling cats, friendly dogs, and the incessant motion of Italian children, who never seem to go to bed. The chic of Italian restaurants, like their food and most of the conversation, never loses a down-to-earth quality.

I adore this aspect of Roman life. I would not trade the warmth, confusion, and relaxed atmosphere of an Italian trattoria for the best restaurants in the world. It is exciting to go to a snob, gourmet restaurant once in a while. But give me the inexpensive trattoria for regular fare. The food is simple and substantial and has color. The service, even when slow, is well-intentioned. There is a smell of herbs. Everyone looks marvelous, because everyone, clearly, is enjoying himself. There is no exact equivalent abroad. French provincial restaurants come closest. In the States, one only finds the same feeling when a group of friends gathers at someone's house for an informal evening. Americans excel at organizing informal dinners at home, but in Rome, this is true primarily in the art world. And as long as the trattoria institution lasts, Romans will eat out.

Who can resist a little Roman beach restaurant off-season? You sit there in a blissful daze from the sun and wine, fingers sticky from broiled prawns. You go for a walk on the deserted beach, stick a toe in the freezing water, stop for a coffee to pick you up, and drive back in a half hour to town. That beats any cure at a beauty salon.

Should fashion revert to Rubens' ladies, I am afraid I could pick up the necessary bulk in a week. I like to eat: sauces, those divine salamini, wild boar, broiled mushrooms, baby lamb, pork with fennel. Surely, a woman's warmth and charm depend on at least a minimum of self-indulgence. Drink that wine, eat that pasta!

But you cannot do it every day and happily, I tell myself, you get to the point where it does not matter. If you practice discipline, the tummy gets the message and shrinks. Let's face it, it's better when you eat simply and just a little. You do not feel deprived.

I am against real dieting unless it is planned for individual need and supervised by a doctor. For taking off a few pounds, the secret is and always has been to eat less, keep the proteins, vitamins, minerals, fats, and carbohydrates balanced, and eliminate the gooey enchantments.

Italians in Rome and Florence with weight problems are beginning to go to Dr. Fulvio Rossi, an endocrinologist and gerentologist with offices in both cities. While slimming his patients, Dr. Rossi does not pretend to make them young again, only to slow down the ravages of aging. His cure consists of twelve to fifteen intravenous feedings, at a rate of three a week, of what he describes as biological and biochemical products to disintoxicate the body, especially the liver, as well as additives of trace minerals and non-fattening vitamins. During the first week, the patient only eats hulled wheat and apples and may drink black coffee.

Gradually, potatoes, vegetables, and meat are added.

Most people I know with real reducing problems take them to Rome's Salvador Mundi clinic where the late Dr. A. T. W. Simeon's method is practised. His 500-calorie-per-day diet is uncompromising. One friend of mine discovered she even had to give up her face cream. Absorbed by the skin, it showed up on the scale during her daily weigh-in. One makes the daily trek to the hospital because the strict calorie count is only part of the cure. It is combined and, according to the doctor, is only effective with daily injections for a month of Human Chorionic Gonadotrophin (HCG), a substance extracted from the urine of pregnant women.

The doctor came upon HCG treating "fat boy" patients suffering from Froehlich's syndrome. These are boys with breasts, large hips and buttocks, and underdeveloped genitals. In addition to helping normal sexual development, the injections caused a loss in appetite and a change in shape. The abnormal fat deposits moved.

"Massage, exercising, or dieting alone are not the cure for obesity," the doctor claimed, "because the body always takes back its needed reserves and the excess, abnormal fat is not burned until the dieter is weak and wrinkly." What he means here is the classic plight of the dieter whose face looks like a prune and whose behind is like an elephant's. He said that the combination of HCG and a 500-calorie diet allows the body to consume abnormal fat as food, then stabilizes the weight. (Also, after puberty, HCG has no sexual effect. It is not a sex hormone.)

One of the late Dr. Simeon's most attractive patients was Val Cook, wife of *Newsweek*'s former Rome bureau chief, Philip S. Cook. Val, a cool collected beauty, is tall and slender. To all appearances, she never had a weight problem in her life. But her grandmother was an enormously overweight woman. Val, who had been hefty as a girl, lost weight after her third child. When she put on ten pounds in Rome, she was haunted by visions of fat reaching down at her through the generations.

"I'm a living example of the cure," she said, "Phil thinks it's a bit scary that you've got that stuff running around in your system forever. The point is it works—I lost and I haven't regained. I can take a drink without putting on weight—something I could never do before. I have lots of willpower, but really I wasn't that hungry during the cure. When we were invited out to dinner, I used to take my little doggy bag of diet food along with me."

I think I would have the willpower, too. I just keep hoping I will not have the problem, as long as I eat sensibly. I do not feel smug about it, mind you. In many cases, staying thin is a matter of constitutional luck. There are people for whom two extra shakes of salt equal a pound.

What does intrigue me is the discipline of natural foods as a way of preserving beauty. Unfortunately, Rome is not a health food center, and devotion becomes an import operation. There are a few health food stores in Rome, understocked by international standards, and one macrobiotic shop.

The Italian idea of health food, rather than yeast or wheat germ, is unadulterated wine and olive oil, country ham and salami, fresh truffles, hand-picked mushrooms, homemade bread, and so on. It is a lovely idea, and I would not quarrel with it, except that most of these delights are on their way to extinction.

Angi Rossi, of the Munemann family, now married to Rome life, imports her special foods by the carload from Germany. These include yeast pills, Norwegian algae, pine honey "from Christmas trees," a juice concentrate from seventeen kinds of plants; Fruchtzucker, a very white, very powdery, sweet fruit sugar, and "Granaton." The latter is fermented wheat germ in liquid form. Angi says, "It contains vitamins B, C, I, P, and E, and I feel it's stimulating sexually and you can drink as much as you like. My grandmother always drank it."

Another true believer is Talitha Getty, who explains that she became interested because her husband, Paul, is a health freak. They drink carrot juice by the gallon, dote on yoghurt and Bircher-muesli, use only rock salt, wild or unpolished rice, and brown sugar. Better still, they substitute honey for sugar whenever possible. In Rome, Talitha grows herbs on the terrace, including mint for tea. "For a while, I became a vegetarian like Paul," she said. "It works for him, but I had to give it up. It made me grossly fat." (I might add that I tried it too, at one point, and it made me grossly anemic.)

Talitha buys some of the products locally. Usually she stocks up in Baker Street in London, except for vegetarian pâté, ham, and bacon that, to meet her standards, come from Holland.

Many Romans do swear by honey, perhaps because it is so much in the Mediterranean tradition. It is said to improve stamina (Sir Edmund Hillary took it with him while climbing Mount Everest) and to boost virility (have heard of no outstanding exploits here). I get my honey from the Marquis Gallarate Scotti who has land south of Rome. Other addicts search out hive owners in Calabria where the honey smells of bergamot.

Trying to organize the natural food life in Rome takes dedication, but it is worth it. The lesson here is always the same, whether it's supervised dieting, special treatments, or health foods: You have to want to try them—you have to work at them for them to work for you. Disciplining yourself, caring enough can go a long way toward keeping you young and attractive. Two weeks of discipline and dedication and you can find the right formula. Read, probe, experiment, try!

3 Putting on Your Best Face

There is a theory that age shows first on the elbows, but who really cares that much about a wrinkle on the elbow? Age strikes hardest, fastest, and most disturbingly always at the face and neck, and unless a woman takes to wearing veils, there is no way to hide a face.

"It's the bones that make a face," says Sophia Loren, who happens to have some of the best around. "Without their foundation the house collapses." Sophia, unfortunately, is absolutely right. A durable face depends to a great degree on luck. One either has good bones or one does not. Furthermore, given the same care, some skin types last longer than others, and skin type depends on lucky genes. The pale, transparent porcelain skin of the North—often the most admired—is also the most fragile and needs many times the protection from sun, wind, and cold that other skin types require. Olive skin holds a lot longer, and black ("is beautiful") holds its beauty best of all. Many a Brazilian woman owes her glorious skin to Negro ancestors, and almost any woman looks decidedly better with a slight tan.

Although skin is fragile, much can be done to keep a face going before the sag must either be lifted or lived with. When you cut down on cigarettes (or stop smoking completely) it is amazing how much the skin clears. I used to blame a rather

olive drab skin tone on my Calabrian forebears until I discovered that the olive drab came straight
from a bottle; for me less liquor meant a pinker,
clearer complexion. No one knows about the effect
of drugs, although it is obvious that getting hung
up on anything is no good for beauty.

Men often tell you the best thing for skin is making love. I cannot say I have always found the
quality of *their* skin to be convincing evidence.
The idea of therapeutic sex strikes me as rather
dreary. One goes to bed with a man because of
desire that may also be love, not for health and
pink cheeks. I grant that no sex is a bore, but I
remember a friend woefully telling me of a time
when she had sex three times a day and everything, including her looks, went downhill. The relationship was a mess and no amount of sheer sex
could counteract the strain.

Nervous tension shows up instantly in the face.
When I am nervous, for example, my pores dilate.
When I am in love and being cared for, my face
brightens. But you cannot work in big cities today
without nervous tension and loneliness part of the
time and you have to learn to live with it and
relax.

After business trips and the irregular hours and
food they entail, like many women I take a mas-
sive vitamin cure. When my skin gets too dry, vitamin F99 is invaluable. I also take liver injections
every two months. The injections are often pre-
scribed for people who suffer from cirrhosis of the
liver. Happily, that is not my problem; I take them
because they smooth my skin. Such preoccupation
with the liver is typically Latin, but there is no

doubt in my mind that the state of the liver and the state of the skin are linked.

After trips to New York, I go for two or three facials in a row. Much as I love New York plumbing, I could do without that excessive central heating; it eats up every cream I put on my skin. Normally, I use either foundation or moisturizer. In New York, I use both. My skin is always either dry or dirty, because the heat makes the makeup penetrate too much.

Roman apartments in old palazzi with their big rooms and high ceilings often are too cold. Even in my modern apartment, I supplement the central supply with an electric heater in the bedroom. The farther south in Italy, the worse it becomes, as thousands of Americans who have frozen in "sunny" Sicily can attest. Personally, I would rather put on an extra sweater and save my skin—at least, that is what I tell myself on the chillier days.

A balanced diet also helps skin tone because it affects you from inside out. In my case, balanced means including meat. The vegetarian approach that many beauties use interests me in theory but, in practice, it makes me anemic. An occasional fast day—once every two weeks—confining myself to mashed potatoes and camomile tea, for example, brightens the skin while keeping weight down.

At a certain age, however, the belief that one can never be thin enough can spell disaster to a face that needs a few extra body pounds to plump it up and keep it smooth. As one of Rome's more dashing men once confessed in chagrin: "My dear, at a certain age, you have to choose. It's either the face or the behind that stays up."

Sports, walking, and all exercise lend extra radiance to the skin. The yoga headstand, in particular, is excellent for the complexion. (Unfortunately, I cannot stand on my head—I get up all right but then come crashing down. Since I am a perfectionist and hate to do things unless I can do them well, I have all but abandoned yoga.) In similar fashion, the "bicycle exercise"—lying on the floor, then swinging the legs and hips up in the air supported by the hands, and pedaling the legs—brings blood rushing to the face. The laziest way to achieve the same effect is simply to stretch out supine and relax with your feet up on pillows.

Here are some of my favorite exercises for keeping the face up. Some of them are based on yoga, some are not:

1. Touch your chin to your chest, then roll your head all the way around in a circle, alternately clockwise and counterclockwise.

2. Hold your head up, chin high, then swing your head first to the left shoulder and then to the right. At shoulder position, lean the head so that your ear almost touches your chest, and then lean the other way so that the opposite ear almost touches the back.

3. Bring your lower lip as close to your nose as possible, count three and release.

4. Repeat the lip movement, but while the lip is up, shift the mouth to the left, then right.

All of these exercises are excellent for the neck and the lower part of the face, as is the simple trick of remembering throughout the day to keep the chin up—it pulls the neck out. For the vertical lines that form between the brows, exercising by wrinkling the nose hard is the best antidote.

The beauty secret in outdoor sports, along with the charge they give to circulation, is perspiration. Consuelo Crespi observes that girls are never more glowing than when they have just come off the tennis courts and have had a shower. Any of you who play tennis know the feeling and the look.

There is only one precaution to take with the outdoor life, but it is essential. The face should never, never be overexposed to the sun. If you must stretch out and bake—not the greatest for body skin either—the face must be reasonably well protected.

Former international model and photographer Buxy Gancia is always slightly tanned. A tall, slender blonde, Buxy leads a country life in her house near Lausanne. But she dons enormous goggles to protect her face when skiing and wears big hats by the lake or sea. Marella Agnelli puts face screening on her frugal beauty-care list, although her skin is somewhat dark and could take more sun than most.

One of the most talented young makeup artists, Gil of Max Factor, says that too much sun makes you look older in more ways than one. It ages and tends to wrinkle the skin, causing permanent damage. Too much sun and sea irritates the eyes and you spend all evening dabbing at the corners. Too deep a tan also adds years because the harsh contrast in color makes the eyes look tired. He refers, of course, to eyes that normally go with a paler look; Blacks have eyes that harmonize with their dark skin.

For protection during midsummer when the sun is strongest, I try to keep my face in the shade. Last year in Sardinia, where we all ended up nude on a deserted beach, I put my bikini on my face.

Lots of women believe in ointments and oils, but I do not like the feel of them and get the impression that they make the face fry. After a day in the sun, however, a moisturizing mask calms the skin. I also recommend using a very strong night cream if one has been out skiing or sunning all day.

My plan is to try to keep some color all year round. Unfortunately, I do not have much time in the winter to get away to the mountains. So it is nice to live in Rome where one can come home for lunch and a sunbath at the window.

Cristina Ford throws caution to the winds and is the outstanding exception to the moderate sun rule. I have never seen her without a tan. She absolutely soaks up the sun, follows it, worships it— and looks glorious. On the Mediterranean, she is up on deck sunning all day. In Grosse Pointe, she uses a sun reflector at the window. She changes creams to protect her face and body. The sun may dry out most skins, but not hers. Even in the city, she always has a moist, healthy, lusty look.

On a cruise last summer, she had the great sense to use no makeup at all. At the beginning of the cruise, the other women did. Then they confined its use to evening—and finally, following her lead, they gave it up. She made them look overdone. The year she showed up in Capri dressed in well-cut shirts and jeans, everyone in more elaborate turnouts looked too contrived. Of course, Cristina looks so marvelous in jeans because she is small-boned and slender. There is a good curve of bosom, but almost no hips, and long, long legs. The truth is that anything she does is contagious. She was not the first woman in Detroit to have her hair streaked, but after she did it, there were many more streaked blondes in Detroit.

As one admirer enthuses, Cristina is a great export. Without even trying, she seems to say: "I am Italian, copy me." It is her directness and refreshing simplicity that influence people, and these are qualities that even Italians often lose. What a smile Cristina has! It is a smile that lights up a room. She has always abhorred pretense and pomposity of any kind. Her standard answer to bores and snobs is: "I don't know about you. I was raised on bread and onions."

Cristina may be an exception to the moderate-sun principle, but what she and every woman must respect in basic skin care is cleansing. It used to infuriate me years ago when one of my friends, who had flawless skin, confessed that sometimes when she was very tired and got in late, she slept with her makeup on and took it off in the morning. Maybe in your twenties you can get away with it. I never could, and no one can for long.

There are two schools of cleansing: the soap and water school and the milk and cream school. I happen to belong to the former, making sure only that the soap itself is creamy and mild. Veruschka and Consuelo Crespi also are confirmed soapers. New York's Dr. Lazlo turned them on. Marella Agnelli, who only uses pharmaceutical cosmetics, prefers both an inalterable cold cream and a non-soap soap.

Pharmaceutical brands are now much in vogue in Italy. Inexpensive, and sold only in drugstores, they doubtless were discovered first by young girls and women on a budget. But models, actresses, and sophisticates, who love to change and experiment, soon followed. Sophia Loren, since the birth of Carlo, Jr., uses Johnson's Baby Oil. It cannot be pure coincidence that both Virna Lisi and Talitha Getty are onto "Vichy" cleansing milk. They travel in different circles, but all their friends have in common a gift for sleuthing out new products and trends. With a new backer, French Vichy, long associated with mineral water, has suddenly found itself with a "sleeper" in its beauty products—until the vogue for pharmaceuticals passes, replaced by something else.

Minor skin problems fall into two categories: those caused by an excess of oils in the skin, and those caused by the absence of those same oils. Below are some of my favorite kitchen recipes for coping with one or the other of these difficulties:

For an excellent astringent mask, plop the yolk of an egg into a cup, add a shake of olive oil and a few drops of lemon juice, smear on the face (taking care to avoid the delicate skin around the eyes), and while it pulls, rest with your feet higher than your head.

An alternate, the rage a few years ago with the chic Paris homosexuals, is this: Take the white of one egg, a teaspoon of the best olive oil, beat, and apply for 20 minutes. Remove with hot face towel, lace trim optional.

Still another mask consists of one tablespoon of lanolin and one teaspoon of Balsam of Peru, mixed until smooth. If made in larger quantities, the mixture should be kept in an airtight jar. The mask is left on the face for 5 minutes.

Glycerine and honey are venerable moisturizers. Water in which the roots or leaves of comfrey have been distilled or warmed olive or almond oil are said to combat wrinkles. (Dried comfrey may be used when fresh is not available.) To remove

freckles, cover fresh elder flowers with cold distilled water and allow to stand overnight. Strain,
and wash your face with the water in which the
flowers were steeped. I do not see why anyone
would want to remove freckles, maybe because I
have never had any.

Sweet almond oil, applied before washing the
face, counteracts dryness of skin. Milk curdled
with lemon cleanses the skin, but use it fast before it smells.

Many of these old formulas have been incorpo-
rated into contemporary ready-mades, easy to obtain and to apply. I think that the value of these
older ways is that they force you to take time to
look beautiful. When all you have to do is dip into
a jar, you expect instant beauty and tend to grow
lazy. When you mix your own mask, on the other
hand, you have to be attentive to make sure that
it will come out right. Having made this effort,
you apply it with more care and watch the effect
more eagerly. It is this attentive attitude that
counts, and if using old recipes can teach it, by
all means get back into the kitchen.

But for really troubled skin, the only wisdom
lies in taking it to a specialist. And since not even
specialists are infallible, one may have to consult
more than one, or find oneself in Talitha Getty's
situation. Talitha first went to a specialist as a preventive measure. Her skin was doing nicely, but
she thought it might do better.

"He was one of those water freaks," she said,
"a true believer in soap and water and absolutely
mad for purity. Astringent had to be purest alcohol. The only trouble was that the brand of prod-

ucts that he thought were the purest were poison to me. In three months, I broke out in rampant acne." Talitha, who had not had problems before, decided to cure herself by a process of elimination. First she threw out the specialist's prescriptions, then she carefully experimented with other products until she found the ones that were right. She was her own best authority. Unless a skin condition is serious, a woman's curiosity and will to experiment may be all the expertise she needs.

Once one has done what one can for the skin, exercised the face muscles to keep them toned, and realized how much or how little one's particular set of bones can be relied on, makeup can serve as an almost endless resource. But cosmetics alone do not beautify. What is needed is that old loving care in using them and a critical eye toward that familiar image in the mirror. Cosmetics can do wonders or wreak horrors, and one can spend years learning all the tricks only to discover that the less done the better. The point here is that simplicity is the result of knowledge, not the lack of it.

The decision of what is to go on your face is further complicated by the fact that fashion in faces now changes as rapidly as it does in clothes. I thought I knew a year ago what was best for my own style. But what I and many other women were doing suddenly seemed old hat, and we all had to find a new "best." There is no longer only one way to put on makeup any more than there is only one way to dress. This gives you the freedom to put forth the face you prefer and, at the same time, adds to the general confusion. It leaves the woman who wants to look as attractive as possible but who simply does not have the time or inclination to spend much time in front of the mirror in something of a quandary.

There is one shining anchor in the contemporary flux: All of the formerly "official" canons of beauty are now obsolete except possibly the belief that imperfection and "wrong" proportion are more interesting than classic harmony. Few of us could ever be classic beauties. Almost all of us have a defect to play up or hide. Makeup expert Gil, for example, adores both Sophia Loren and Twiggy precisely because he says everything is wrong with them—they have a thousand defects and the intelligence to make their own style.

Gil confesses that dealing with ugly women destroys him; he only thrives with beautiful people. But he means beauty in the larger sense—that includes the right physical attributes, but also the right charm, the right intelligence, the right sense of who one is and what life one leads. "I hate makeup," he exclaims. "Look at that woman over there—her makeup is impeccable and totally wrong. Who knows how long she spent on it, but it isn't her. Anything goes now, but what goes best on most women is a casual look, the hair pulled back in a chignon or tied with a ribbon, lip gloss, gloss on cheekbones, a glow to the eyes, as if they didn't have time to do anything more. They did, of course, but they knew when to stop."

According to Gil, even the old divisions between day and evening looks, between outdoor and indoor makeup have blurred. Beauty is psychology, being one's type. And if one's type is mysterious and cosmetically complex, that implies the leisure to indulge it. There is no sense trying to be mysterious when you spend most of your waking life in an office. In that case, forget all the lashes and liner—you can and should have another kind of attraction.

Rino Carboni, who did the fabulous makeup for Fellini's *Satyricon,* among other films, has a more radical approach. Along with his movie work, Carboni has done makeup on department store customers, so he speaks with a knowledge of real women as well as of fantasy creatures. "A makeup man who says 'I'll transform you' is stupid," he claims. "A woman wants to be either herself or what she thinks of as her better self. If you're an actress or a model, photogenic quality is all-important and you have to have a face that looks well in almost any circumstance and that a majority of people will like.

"But other women have a choice. They have to be aware of their defects, but it's either to diminish them or to bring them out. In other words, a woman can try to be more attractive in the accepted sense or she can try to be unique. If she has to please only herself and the few people she cares about, she might be wise to expose that vast forehead and play it up with makeup instead of hiding it. She could flaunt that irregular nose or chin. What she would achieve would be the one face in a crowd, because it would be her own face unabashed."

Carboni is aware that most of us cannot go around looking like portraits or paintings of creatures from *Satyricon.* He suggests a compromise: By day we look as conventionally attractive as possible; at night, without inhibitions, we unwrap our real face or create the face of our aspirations.

For Carboni, beauty is being true to type, not stereotype. Making defects work for you, however, is a difficult art. The experts argue that Sophia Loren is one of the few who mastered it. When Sophia was an aspiring actress, she was told that, with her profile, she could never be a movie star. Sophia refused to have her nose changed and learned to make up her eyes instead. In time, women with more regular features wished they had hers and tried in vain to imitate them.

But not all irregularities can result in striking beauty. Many women, including myself, have had defects they preferred to camouflage or eliminate rather than emphasize. When the choice is between looking like a character study or being as pretty and attractive to men as possible, I am for women who opt for the latter.

Carboni's great value is that he is endlessly creative. His makeup work, whether it intensifies or beautifies, is a source of provocative ideas. One should remember that he started in the theater, where faces have to project. He has never lost a love of masks and dramatic effects. It is the anomaly in a face that interests him. I go along when he talks in terms of contrast in shape and lines, something that any woman should study in her mirror. For example, if one has a round face, small features, and round eyes, a divergent line is needed somewhere. Straight eyebrows perhaps—certainly not eyebrows in rounded curves like the rest of the face. Conversely, angular shapes need to be offset by roundness. The makeup of eyes, cheeks, or mouth could supply it.

Carboni says that we look at a face as we read a page, starting at the upper left side. The trick is to provide interest that stops the gaze from going from eyebrow down the nose and out of the face. Particularly, as we grow older, attention should be centered on the up planes. Makeup and hair should go against the force of gravity that is pulling the face down.

Here I would add that one of the few basic rules in makeup is to go lighter as you grow older. A face-lift can rejuvenate, but heavy pancake on top of it adds the fifteen years the surgeon removed. The other rule, to my mind, is that being slightly plain is better than being horribly made-up. Even with little effort, most women get by all right during the day. Comes the big night, although out of practice in glamour, they strive for the dream effect and cannot carry it off. I understand why Carboni encourages women to let out all the stops at night and become their secret aspiration, but perhaps because I am a woman and have experimented myself, I know that to do so takes infinite sophistication.

If your life-style is casual, add a few eyelashes and maybe a hairpiece after dark and forget the exotic endeavors. In fact, forget all the extras if you are going to be touching them all night to make sure they are still in place. When one of the kings of Naples was asked to approve the new dress uniforms for his troops, he answered, "Dress them any way you want—they'll still run away." In other words, if you are not a militant beauty at heart, you will not act like one despite the trimmings.

I worked for over a year and a half for Eve of Roma until the company's assets were sold. While she lived, Eve Elmes was her own best advertisement. After her sudden death in 1968, other women were needed to personify her products. Eve was a woman of great spirit, one of the last *grandes dames* of the beauty business. She thought it unforgivable in a woman not to look after her face as soon as she got up and before she did anything else. This could seem a bit steep for a woman dashing to get her husband off to the office or the children off to school. For Eve, it was a matter of habit to be formed and never forsaken. She would rather get up a half hour earlier than be seen as the proverbial unmade bed. On the other hand, she insisted that going to bed with a face smeared with cream is bad for the skin as well as the love life. The night cream she used could be applied for 15 minutes and removed.

Eve was one of the first to suggest pale lipstick, unpopular at the time, and the gleaming, suntanned, natural look. She herself wore little makeup and only had facials when the seasons changed. Even then, she had them primarily to check on the quality of treatment in her salon. She was a great innovator and beauty adviser.

When I traveled on business, I spent several hours every day in department stores as a beauty adviser. I adored this sort of work because I have always had a Pygmalion tendency. If a woman is a nuclear physicist or a doctor, she probably has a completely different outlook on the importance of beauty and no time to waste on Pygmalion intrusions. With the women who came to me in stores, on the contrary, I was free to say what I thought. If they were not looking for advice, they would not have come.

From what I saw, the trouble is that women do

not experiment enough with what they buy, as if putting cash on the line in itself should be enough. Without awareness, without follow-through, cash on the line has never been enough for anything. To illustrate, here are some of my department store experiences:

Instructions for a whitener say to put it under the eyes. One customer asked me if she could continue it up and out a bit farther. "Try it," I said. "If it looks good on you, do it." (Usually, the trick is to put it not on the dark circles under the eyes, which accents them, but on the very top of the cheekbone so that it detracts from the hollow grayness. But it depends on the amount of bag and the facial structure.) As for the woman with a droopy eyelid who wondered whether we might have a cream for it, I told her no, a cream would help only after plastic surgery.

One customer told me she found her moisturizer too greasy for her. When I suggested she use it instead as a night cream, she looked at me in surprise and delight. "Can you?" she asked.

Another found that her base turned slightly gray on her skin. My suggestion was to add a few drops of liquid tan until the mixture comes to the proper glow. To the woman who was unhappy because her Number Three base was too light for her, I suggested that if she bought a Number Five and mixed them, she would have twice the quantity and the right color. If you make a mistake, why not cut the loss instead of starting from scratch? Of course, I am European, which may be why I think that way.

One has to experiment. One has to be curious. This applies even to the use of well-established brands of any beauty product. Why, for example, does Talitha Getty look divine doing her eyes with kohl? Talitha, in her travels, went to North Africa, fell in love with it, and could not discover enough about it. That is why. Kohl recreates for her the excitement a teenager finds with her first eye pencil.

"You can't really get the good stuff here," she says. "Kohl is antimony. In Marrakesh you can see the beautiful silver stones it comes from. Only women past menopause are supposed to grind it. That's to make it more pure. Arab men used to wear it, and it's absolutely safe." Traditionally, kohl is kept in a tiny ivory bottle and applied with a tapered ivory stick. Talitha uses an ivory stick, but her empiricism has led her to substitute a glass phial as a container. Her ivory bottle always leaked when she traveled, which was not very practical.

As I look at the beauties I know, I see that each one has arrived at her style by a process of successive discoveries and elimination. Granted that psychological quirks can enter into the picture, the paring down is anything but artless. Former model Mirella Haggiag is enchanted with the current "unmade-up" approach. She says, "Maybe we'll change again, but when I look at some of my old pictures, I shiver: all the long liner and powder. Now everything is nuance and nature—a good, bright face."

Mirella starts with mascara and moisturizer in the morning, adds eyeliner in the afternoon and "the rest" in the evening—the rest being an eyelash here and there if the evening is important. On dreary winter mornings, she also uses foundation and a drop of liquid rouge.

Sophia Loren excels at all the tricks when she

wants to. They include the instant eye enlargement and lift of surgical tape that pulls the skin up and back between the eye and ear, the tape caught and hidden under the hair. But off work at her villa in the country near Rome, she wears almost no cosmetics—a bit of black makeup for the eyes and a splash of "Joy" for the pleasure.

Virna Lisi, even more beautiful off camera than on, does almost nothing to her face in private life because she finds that working at it too hard brings contrary results. With her classic beauty, less is more. But this also holds true for Marella Agnelli, whose beauty, though extremely thoroughbred, is nonclassic.

Consuelo Crespi, who prefers a more sophisticated appearance, still never looks "made-up." She confesses that for her to achieve what seems almost natural takes behind-the-scenes effort. Consuelo is refreshingly honest: "I like a glowy face. Unless you have very good bone structure, and I don't, the forehead, cheeks, and chin should be a bit shiny, but not the nose. Using tissues designed to prevent shine works better for me than powdering my nose. My daughter puts her makeup on in two minutes; I take twenty-five, and every year, you take five minutes more. But the fatal mistake is to put on more makeup because you look tired."

I am not sure exactly where I fit in. I certainly wear makeup, yet I, too, wear less now than ever before. The one thing I have to do, though the technique may vary, is my eyes. If I do not, it looks as if I forgot to bring them along. When my son, Diego, saw me once at the shore without eye makeup, he told me I looked just like a German nanny. My son, who has lost none of his candor since then, was ten at the time.

Most of us feel "undressed" without some minimum makeup. It used to be lipstick. Now it is mascara or liner or shadow stick because, next to good bone structure and skin tone, the eyes do the most for a face. That does not mean they have to be swimming in makeup. I cannot imagine Marella Agnelli, for one, with false eyelashes. They simply are not her type. And even with eyes, the current trend is away from heavy accent.

After years of liner, now it seems too harsh. The white I used to put over and under the eye last season became a bore. Costume designer Piero Tosi (Visconti's *The Damned*), who always hated visible white highlights, used to call it the "poached egg" look. Instead of liner, I now do shading with gray stick, which is less harsh and, used with mascara, quite sufficient.

Moisturizer and lip gloss are my other products except in winter, when the light on the face changes. Winter usually requires foundation and, for evening, rouge. But never wear foundation when you go to the hairdresser's because sitting under the dryer makes it overpenetrate. Apply the foundation after the hair is done.

I also find that, except in New York or other superheated cities that dry the skin, nourishing cream is needed only where wrinkles tend to form: the outer corners of the eyes, the smile lines, and the throat. The rest of the skin absorbs the cream too much and this makes the pores dilate.

The beauty who has been everywhere and back with makeup is Veruschka, who substituted cosmetics for clothes and launched the nude look a few years back. That was Veruschka of a thousand masks, Veruschka of the long body covered in strategic spangles, striped like a tiger, stenciled like a leopard, painted like a flower.

"Two years ago, I could spend hours in front of a mirror trying colors," she says. "I had fun gluing on strange eyelashes, drawing on designs. My face wasn't a face anymore, it was a shaped canvas. I wanted to bring out everything I had inside so I loved changing makeup or type. I like to look very sexy or very childish (the high, round forehead helps here), like someone in an old painting or like a black girl.

"When I went to Japan for photographs, I studied old prints. The eyebrows were strange and way up high, so I took mine off and made new ones for each picture—just two red points, or all little points, pink and blue eyebrows, just one delicate line higher than usual, then one too low."

Now, in private life, it depends on her mood. Veruschka started applying false eyelashes one by one several years ago. By now it is big business and she doesn't do it anymore. She only puts them at the corners. When she wants big eyes, the liner starts dark and disappears. The rest of the eye is all shading with different browns, lighter to bring out a bone, darker for depth. The idea is great softness and blur as opposed to a line drawing. Her only rule with makeup is that you must be able to "feel" the skin underneath. The essence of Veruschka is change. One day, if she feels like a hard look, she puts it on. That evening she might be soft and feminine, and the next day on the street you see her with no makeup at all. Had she less plasticity of face and whim, she would not have become such a great model. Most of us have to struggle to find one good face and a few variations on our basic theme.

"Ah! Veruschka, how divine," says makeup man Gil. "With Veruschka, anything goes"—and with you what goes and what does not? Have you really taken the time to find out what is you in makeup now, or are you just parroting the ads or an actress whom you like to think looks like you? Do you persist in the illusion that following the same makeup pattern will give you her appeal? Who knows? Maybe you can succeed, but unless you constantly experiment and seek personal advice, you will never learn to create your own best image—and that should be your goal.

4   *Glorious Hair*

Even the least vain woman feels better when her
hair looks right. No matter how intellectual or businesslike, women still inwardly cringe when they
have to keep an impromptu appointment and their
hair is a mess. (You cannot always dash home for
that wig either.) But no Italian woman would
dream of being seen anywhere in rollers. Anywhere
includes the bedroom, if there is a man lurking
about.

As a result, Rome hairdressers are always busy.
They have been since the time of the Caesars.
There are almost as many coiffeurs listed in the
classified pages of the Rome telephone directory as
there are bars and cafés. If one adds men's barbers,
the bars and cafés are outnumbered. One tries to
get appointments during the slack hours, early in
the morning or just after lunch.

Better still, with an active life, one tries to keep
hair so simple that it can be washed at home if
necessary. This tolds true in every city. Unfortunately, not everyone's hair responds well to simplicity. If you have problem hair, even on a tight
beauty schedule, you have to find the time to have
it done professionally, and often.

If it is the hairstyle, not the quality of the hair,
that is complicating life, then a good look at what
most contemporary beauties do may be a basic lesson in strategy. Most of them simplify. They either

wear their hair shoulder-length and straightish, or they wear it short and shaped by cutting.

I used to almost feel undressed without hairpieces. Now I wear my hair loose to the shoulders with sports clothes, or tie it back in a "George" (as in Washington) style. These hairdos are classics and, if they suit the face, have a casual glamour that is very contemporary. No small point in their favor—men always like them.

At this moment, I still own a half-dozen hairpieces and one cheap wig, preserving them for special occasions. Many women swear by wigs, but I, personally, find them rather a bore. At home in Rome, I am organized enough about my hair not to need them; when I am traveling, they are a nuisance because they require a case. Every time real-hair wigs are washed, they have to be set professionally. It gets to the point where you need a Rolls Royce at the door just to ferry your wigs back and forth. Hairpieces can be wound around a magazine or a roll of cotton and then stuffed in a suitcase or a drawer. I prefer to have mine washed at the hairdresser's, but it is not necessary, and they do not have to be set.

When you are trying to learn how to cope with your hair, you should have your hair done by the most talented hairdresser you can find. But remember that putting fragile hair into even the best hairdressing hands is not always a guarantee of success (although there is no better one I can think of). Success comes only with experience. The hairdresser does not always know what your particular head of hair can take, nor do you at first. The first time you go to a top hairdresser, let him do whatever he wants but realize that even then the results may not be fantastic. The first time I went to Alexandre, for example, I came out with a very conventional style. I was far less experienced in hair then than I am now, far less sure of myself in both fashion and beauty. He must have sensed this and, very wisely, played it safe. Also he was not familiar with my hair, nor with me and the life I led.

Years later, Alexandre did my hair for the Rothschild ball at Ferrières. That time the vibrations were right, the magic took place. Maybe I was already a different woman—a more defined personality—and easier to transform. He re-created the Elizabeth of Austria coiffure in the famous portrait by Winterhalter. Her long hair, worn high on the crown, was emblazoned with diamond stars. I had only five stars, and she had many more, but when he had finished, I really felt like an empress.

I would not dream of trying to look that special all the time. I am too busy, and the coiffure would be too elaborate. In a way, it is fortunate that even simpler styles enhanced with hairpieces are now out of fashion for every day wear. Constant use of hair pieces can cause serious scalp problems. Not that I believe for one minute that the return to a more natural look has come about for the good of women's scalps—fashion never changes for such mundane considerations.

On evenings out, as we all know, there is an urge to look more sophisticated and mysterious. That is where the hairpiece comes in. With crepes and chiffons, I still adore to see a mass of hair, real or false, pulled high with the ends dangling. This is a style that may be on its way out, but as far as I am concerned, if it suits me, it is not out yet.

If I have time, I let the hairdresser build the style. If not, I have watched what the experts do and practiced enough at home to pile it up for myself. Relying on someone else is fine, if he is your own personal coiffeur, always at beck and call. Otherwise, any woman is well advised to have a few numbers she can whip up on her own. You learn to arrange hair just as you learn to apply make-up—by observing and experimenting.

If you are using hairpieces often instead of for special occasions and have no problems, fine, but you should be aware of the damage they can do. The Crespis, at one point, were terribly worried when their daughter Pilar's hair began to fall out. She was not yet eighteen. Respite from hairpieces was ordered by her trichologist and that restored her hair. The technique I learned from Alexandre is also a scalp-saver. By the time most hairdressers have clamped in several hairpieces, you are in pain. With Alexandre's technique they do not hurt. He attaches them high on the crown so that they do not pull as much.

Here I should add, in passing, that I have my hair streaked the whitest possible blond once a month—an alternate six- and three-hour process when done properly. I know it is true in many countries, but in Italy where it is rarer, one can never be blond enough. (Hairdressers in Rome use a higher concentration of peroxide than is the custom in the United States.) Needless to say, between the streaking and the effects of hairpiece abuse, I wound up at the local trichologist with scalp troubles of my own.

It was small consolation to discover that Edward Goodman, Rome's leading trichologist, rarely sees a head that has not suffered from willful tampering these days. He is willing to blame some of these problems on busy city life that patients cannot control, but most of the ills of hair and scalp are self-inflicted.

"Hair reflects the way you live," he believes. "Peasants working in the fields have stronger, better hair. So do certain types of manual workers. The reason is less nervous tension."

With some people, nervous tension induces pains in the tummy; with others, the hair falls out. But the principle cause of hair trouble in women, in Mr. Goodman's experience, is not stress; it lies in overuse of chemicals, which leads to breakage and all the dreariness of dull, lifeless hair.

Ponytails, if worn constantly, encourage peripheral baldness (alopecia), which sometimes begins to show even in little girls whose hair is always combed that way. Even hair straightening, unless done very skillfully, weakens the hair. Permanents also weaken, especially permanents done on top of coloring.

What was a surprise to me was learning that brushing can be a menace. Mr. Goodman claims that whoever started the notion that a hundred vigorous strokes a day are good for the hair must have died of scalp infection and almost bald. Victorian ladies who observed this dictum reserved a space on their dressing table for hair tidies, little silver or china containers with a hole in the lid where they stuffed the hair that remained in the brush. They then had puffs made from the lost hair to fill in the missing glory.

Mr. Goodman discourages all but the gentlest brushing. A good whack with the brush can scratch the scalp. Any foreign material on the scalp can then enter the scratch and begin infection. For the limited brushing that is necessary, natural bristle brushes are recommended. Combs should have evenly spaced teeth with smooth sides so that they do not catch and break the hair.

Mr. Goodman, incidentally, has gray hair, but plenty of it. He is often called upon to give his verdict on straightening and coloring when a client's hair is difficult. He is an advocate of preventive medicine and now rotates between Eve of Roma's salon and Alba's, the meccas for beautiful people's hair.

Alba has that intensely feminine outlook that the trichologists of this world will simply have to cope with. She is blond—that is, she was born that way and took matters into her own hands when nature changed her into a mouse. So what if her hair is fragile and fine? "I'd rather have only three blond hairs than a crop of chestnut-colored ones," she says, "I loved Diana Vreeland when she told me, 'You're a blonde because your spirit is blond.'"

I am in favor of this spirit. As long as you know the possible risks involved if your hair is not the strongest, why not be any color that suits you and makes you happy? I do not think I shall want to be blond at seventy, but if I am gray and the gray looks terrible with my skin, you can be sure I will not stay gray.

Alba's fame coincided with the vogue for long hair, which they pulled back and piled into extraordinary tails, swirls, and loops. The hair—and innumerable hairpieces—would be caught with bows, jewels, or dangling plastic hoops. Results often were as witty as they were glamorous; for example: the double ponytail, one worn above the other and both cut off straight like paintbrushes, and the horn of plenty with a Christmas tree ball at the tip. And then there was the wired hairpiece that sprang out to form a daisy. . . . All the chic women of Rome wore them.

"But we sensed we had to change," says Alba. "Within ten months after we did short hair and showed it during a Valentino collection, 50 percent of our customers had their hair cut. Long hair and the gypsy look are out. The trend is back to a medium length, worn soft."

But if the demand for hairpieces is in rapid decline, Alba finds the wig industry is as big as ever. Her American clients often walk out with four hundred dollars' worth at a crack. "A woman with fine hair has to have wigs," she says. "So do women who travel and women whose appearance is important in their work. There isn't always time to slip into the hairdresser's—and they're not about to wear curlers to bed!"

Despite my reservations about wigs and my preference, when the mood warrants them, for hairpieces, I agree with Alba about the importance of color. If your own displeases you, change it! The best color depends on your skin. It need not be blond. But the idea is to go light rather than dark. The darker, harsher shades tend to kill any face that was not born with them.

The wrong shape is even worse than the wrong color. I was twenty-eight when back-combing started—with the result that at twenty-eight it was discovered that I had a good profile. My face is narrow, my neck is long and, like most Italians, I have a very defined jawline. Hair swept back and up for height gave my profile the long unbroken line it needed. Suddenly, I was a different, more sophisticated type. I now find that back-combed hair looks better on almost all women.

The same style does not suit everyone, however —that would be too easy. I think the only true test is to take a hard look at the reflection in the mirror, then push your hair around until the best shape emerges.

Sometimes it is easier to spot what is wrong with your hairstyle in examining a snapshot of yourself. Or you may find the answer by looking at photographs of other women with similar facial proportions. Seeing a photograph of someone else with a round face who looks good in bangs, for example, may show you why your own round face looks awful when your hair is pulled straight back.

The one general rule with hairstyles is that when one is over a certain age, hair should be worn short. It may be an optical illusion, but short hair seems to lift the lines of a face better than longer hair. Chignons and twists are an alternative for older women, but only for those who are adept with them and who are blessed with hair that neither draggles nor wisps. And if all that can be achieved is a dreary bun, you might as well cut it off.

To keep it soft and shining, hair should be shampooed every four days, rinsing the hair until it squeaks when squeezed. Vegetable tar shampoos are the best in my experience of all those readily available. But should you, or friends of yours, be going to Morocco, try to get a few bars of *jhassoul*, which is absolutely fabulous.

Jhassoul is made from Moroccan earth and should be diluted with water into a greasy liquid paste before use. You rinse your hair, apply the paste, wait until it dries like mud, then rinse the hair again. As it dries, you begin to suspect *jhassoul* is made from camel dung. It is not, though even if it were, I would use it. The hair comes out so baby-soft and shiny.

The regular shampoo rule applies to dry as well as oily hair, at least in big-city pollution. (You can tell which type you have by the way it looks and feels.) My hair, for instance, would tend naturally to be oily. But now I have had it streaked so much, the problem is dryness. If you have your hair colored, you know exactly what I mean. Unless a conditioner is used after shampooing, the hair feels like straw.

Another help for dry hair is to rub it with linseed oil before you go to bed (wrapping the head in a plastic shower cap to save the pillow case) and to shampoo it first thing in the morning. To save your man, the linseed treatment is only for nights you sleep alone.

One of the first signs of unhealthy hair, apart from lack of luster, is that it will not hold a set or combing. Consultation with a trichologist is in order before worse problems start. On the other hand, dandruff often responds to vitamin F99 without the expense of specialist consultation.

As for split ends, I twist as much hair at a time as will go around a finger, then quickly singe the ends that stick out and will not twist, with a lit candle. The emphasis here is on "quickly"—you do not want to set your hair on fire. The first time I watched a hairdresser do it. When I saw the bill, I decided to do it myself at home.

Of the beauties in this book, some are blessed

and some are damned by hair no matter what they do. Buxy Gancia, tall, slender, and used to casual country or resort life, lets her hair hang straight to her shoulders. She has it streaked professionally, then washes it often herself. She owns a chignon hairpiece for evenings, but most evenings she does not wear it.

Sophia Loren and Virna Lisi simplify, in part out of professional reaction. Sophia's hair, extremely fine, needs constant attention when she is filming. At home, now that it is long, she is only too content to wear it down and forget all the fuss. Virna still recalls a film for which the roots at the part in her hair had to be retouched at seven every morning. Out of sheer exasperation, when the film was over, she marched into her hairdresser's, Alfio and Rossana, and had them cut her hair as short as possible. She almost had it shaved. Her blond hair is shoulder-length now. She, too, follows the contemporary independent pattern. Except for coloring at the hair dresser's, she can take care of her hair by herself—and prefers to.

Virna has a classically beautiful face, so when she is not wearing her hair down, she can afford to pull it back in the smallest, flattest chignon. That is the way she wore it to a Monte Carlo gala where most of the women showed up with elaborate hairdos. "You know what I mean," she said, "the kind that are so contrived you want to give them a good yank. All night, people kept asking me who had designed my hair because they found it so chic. I had—and it took me ten minutes."

Again, you must realize that it takes Virna ten minutes to arrange her hair only because she has had over fifteen years of schooling in beauty care.

She began to act at age thirteen, and an actress must learn to be clever with her makeup and hair. To varying degrees, we all must. I might add that you do not have to be a classic beauty to wear a chignon. Many faces benefit from its simplicity, and if, on the other hand, it makes you look like a schoolmarm, your mirror will tell you fast enough.

For Marella Agnelli, hair is a painful subject only because "no one can cut except Alexandre— or maybe Kenneth." When it is cut short and properly—the ends flipped up off her face and the nape covered—she washes it herself or slips into salons where she can be out in a half hour. She has worn much the same cut for years. It suits her and suits her life with a man who both loves style and hates any waste of time. I cannot imagine any woman making Gianni Agnelli wait because she is late at the crimper's.

Brunette Mirella Haggiag, after a short haircut at Alba's six months ago, has changed type completely. It is amazing what a new hairstyle can do. "I used to live with toupees," she says, "be photographed with what must have been forty hairpieces at a time. Now they just look fake to me. In the summer at Porto Rotondo, I can't bear all those terrifying women with toupees or terry turbans trying to look divine. I don't wear jewelry anymore. I suppose I'm reacting to a haircut, but I feel I'm myself now. Before, I was a construction job."

Not everyone can solve their problems so easily. Veruschka, who likes lots of "messy hair, moving hair, not that stiff thing," found that hers had started to break. This may be due, in part, to all the working over it is subjected to in modeling, but basically it is a question of fragile hair. Verushka compromises: On the one hand she keeps it long; on the other, she goes regularly to a trichologist to have it treated.

Talitha Getty's hair is very fine, and she likes it shoulder-length. One of the most famous Rome salons permed it, colored it, and then for a magazine spread coiffed it in the tiniest, tightest plaits. It fell out by the clump. Her solution was to cut it short and wait until it grew out healthy again.

Consuelo Crespi is clever with hair, she complains, only because hers is so bad, she has to be. "I'm saved by hairpieces and wigs. Fifteen years ago they didn't exist. It was damn good timing." Her theory is that Americans have better legs, but Italians have healthier hair. She attributes it to climate and the ubiquitous olive oil in the diet.

Consuelo has her hair washed every four days, and often slips into Alba's to have it combed before she goes out for the evening. This is more time than most women are willing to devote to their hair, but it is neither in her nature, nor in the nature of her job as a fashion editor, to look unkempt, hair problem or no hair problem. When swimming, she never wears a bathing cap (remember, the trick here is to rinse the salt water out of the hair right away) but just slips her hair into an elastic band while it dries or ties a scarf around it, letting the ends float free.

Women are not the only ones who have to cope with their hair. Men's can be just as difficult as women's, and even without the threat of incipient baldness, men are vain about their hair. Longer hair for men has only intensified a problem that was already acute. The drama of a barbershop debate over three hairs more or three hairs less at the sideburns or the nape of the neck surpasses any female hysteria at the coiffeur's.

Nino Cerruti solves his hair problems by the do-it-yourself method. For the past year he has been cutting his own hair with one of those special combs available at international pharmacies. The long-handled comb has normal teeth on one side and a cutting edge on the other.

One of Rome's most famous and attractive jewelers washes his hair at home every day, then sits under the dryer to read the papers. When he travels, the dryer travels with him. He is not the type to resort to a toupee should he grow bald, but he aims to defend what he has till the last.

Asked how he cared for his hair, a Roman businessman said he washed it at home. "I wash it every two days. I like the sides flat, so I put on a net before I dry it. Don't write this down, I'll sound ridiculous." Reassured his name would not be mentioned, he continued, "You know the kind of net I mean. You tie it under the chin so it doesn't slip. The net doesn't cover the top, just the sides. I like the top to be full."

Neither the jeweler nor the businessman have any need to be embarrassed. A man's hair has to be washed often, and if it is long, it has to be shaped. Amleto, twenty-three years a Roman barber, gives the same basic advice to actors and bankers. "Wash your hair often, even once a day," he says, "but wash it 'badly.' What I mean is give it a good rinse, but go light with the shampoo."

As for baldness, once it happens, Amleto believes that the only cure is a hair transplant. Keeping hair short does not prevent baldness; growing it long does not provoke it. He does not know about short beds, but blaming the Army helmet you used to wear is ridiculous—ditto the motorcyclist's crash helmet.

Amleto, who has a good head of hair, sees nothing unattractive about men who lose theirs. He finds a bald head much more attactive than a toupee that never fools anyone. Some fashions are charming because they are so obviously fake. The problem with the toupee is that no one is supposed to notice that it is false—and everyone always does.

Really long, hippie hair is now out for men, but the influence lingers on. Sideburns prosper in Rome, half of the ear is still covered, and the nape of the neck is never bare. Male customers frequently describe the good cut they saw on a woman and ask Amleto to imitate it. This is less extreme than it sounds. If a man's hair is hand-dried, a clever barber shapes it as he dries it, with exactly the same technique that is used on women's short hair.

A good cut is done with scissors, a technique that many women's hairdressers seem to have forgotten—to their convenience, not to the customer's. I do not wear my hair short, but women who do have learned the truth about razor cuts, much to their regret. One slip of the razor and you wait three weeks for the "hole" in the air to grow out. Even without mishap, the hair, which may look fine the first day and even the second, has no body. Old-fashioned snipping takes away less and leaves a good mass, however short.

As the distinctions between male and female beauty needs blur, a double trend emerges: Chic women's hairdressers are opening departments for men. The male vanity has come out in the open, and the men want pampering. On the other hand, women with short hair are turning to barbers the way they turn to tailors for made-to-order pants.

5   Have a Lift

Coco Chanel, already in her eighties when asked about cosmetic surgery, remarked that if she ever thought she needed it, she certainly would have it done. Good for Chanel!

If a woman feels happy with the state of her skin, why have it overhauled? Both Jeanne Moreau and Anna Magnani have said they would not part with the bags under their eyes. They believe in letting the years show—the bags are part of their appeal and attest to a heap of living. Elizabeth Taylor also considers every wrinkle a part of her life and wants her life to show.

Not every woman, however, is anxious to have her life show in such detail, especially right up there on her face. One remembers, for example, the tragedy of the Countess of Castiglione, mistress of Napoleon III and a woman whose charm and beauty had changed the face of Europe. At thirty-nine, the countess triple-locked herself into a dimly lit Paris apartment with no mirrors rather than reveal her beauty in decline. Today, if she cared so much about her looks, the countess would not have to become a recluse. She would take hormones, do exercises, and have her face lifted. If she hid at all, it would be from time to time at beauty farms, and it would not be for long.

I happen to believe in preventive cosmetic surgery, in having a little tuck taken in here and there before the face really goes. The point is that today women have a choice about the way they are going to look. To me, the critical moment for most women is sometime in their forties. They have watched the first wrinkles appear and seen the first slack. The chin and throat are not quite what they used to be. But all in all, they are still good-looking, vital, and desirable. Then one day, perhaps because they are over-tired, anxious about work or just depressed because the sky is gloomy, they look in the mirror and a frightening apparition looks back.

Suddenly, the looks have gone, and you have to choose. You want to be beautiful in the objective sense, with the beauty that no one fails to notice, envy, or admire. When you have it, men turn to look in the street. Often their appraisals are offensive, if harmless, and you could do without them— until they stop.

More to the point, you hate what you, yourself, see in the mirror and therefore show to husband, lover, friends, children, colleagues, competitors. If you are a perfectionist, if beauty means being smooth, fresh, and taut, you go to the plastic surgeon.

The other choice is to wait it out. The forties will be rocky, but productive. You want to stay in shape, but exceptional beauty was never your forte. You opt for the strong face, the interesting face. It will not be "beautiful people," but it could be Cartier-Bresson. The ingenue roles, the femme fatale leads are over. It is time to play the character part, if you have it in you. Once past fifty or sixty, a good face, in any sense, is hard to find.

Yankee Katherine Hepburn, the essence of honesty, is remarkable. One of the strongest, most polished faces in New York belongs to *Vogue*'s editor-in-chief, Diana Vreeland. Janet (Genêt) Flanner, Paris correspondent for *The New Yorker*, is extraordinary, with her thatch of hair and proudness of nose and chin. Even homeliness can take its revenge. Eleanor Roosevelt, in her later years, had a face of such character and strength, it was, in its own way, beautiful. We all know women of such style and charm in their unabashed fifties that younger beauties become insipid in their presence.

The forties are the difficult years because you are suspended between two roles. With the active, public life that women lead now, the forties face is unfair. It is too early to grow old gracefully and too late to keep up with the girls.

I remember riding once in Virginia with a glorious woman who was past sixty. As two men went galloping by, tall in the saddle, with much dash and great panache, she said: "The years may bring wisdom, but do you know, desire never dies." In the forties, this feeling is even more acute, and the decline of beauty brings on fits of rage and depression. If you can shed five or ten years, for heaven's sake, do it. Even an eye-lift can make an enormous change.

Clare Booth Luce in New York ran into a younger friend whom she had not seen for several years. After they had greeted each other, Mrs. Luce said: "I know you think I've had my face done, and if you're thinking about it, young lady, you'd better have it done now."

Like most women, I have always been afraid of wrinkles and lines. My approach is to get at them before they really dig in. People less critical than I might not notice them, but I see smile lines, a crinkle at the eye, and already I have visions of a face that hangs down to my ankles.

A lift is done only because old vanity is screaming. No one should decide about these things except yourself. No plastic surgery in itself will get you a man or hold the one you have. Remember that the signs of aging that disturb a woman do not always disturb a man. They can even be erotic as long as the basic rapport is right. Usually when a mature man chases those "fresh young things," their appeal to him goes beyond the fresh young face and body to the youth of the psyche. And then, too, a woman I know had her face lifted and proceeded to have a new affair; it turned out to be such a wretched one that it aged her at least fifteen years.

"It's the old story about the lady who had her breasts done and nobody cared," says Gore Vidal. "Actually, women change their bodies not so much to attract men as to confound other women with their ability to show off clothes."

Obviously, what he is referring to here is not the face, but breast, buttocks, and abdominal lifts. Often, they are done to wear those nothing bikinis rather than clothes. And I would not exclude their being done for sex; it is better than having to turn the lights off every time.

Mostly, it is breast surgery, either lift or reduction of size, that is done as much for clothes as for having a pretty bosom. I did not realize this for years. When you go through a protracted flat puberty as I did, you assume that every woman wants more rather than less bosom. I even tried Niehan's-type cell implants that a Roman doctor had found successful in enlarging eighteen-year-olds' breasts. Perhaps because I was older than that, they did nothing. As many women have discovered, the birth control pill can be a boon to breast development at first, but I found that in time I reverted right back to pre-pill dimensions.

Two Roman beauties I know who have had their breasts lifted were astounded I should ever have wanted larger measurements. Both of them had developed precociously and abundantly, and both were furious that their surgeons had not reduced as well as remolded them. "Luciana, you're out of your mind," one of them said. "Clothes look so much better without a lot of bosom. You get that heavenly long line." At least the two beauties had gone to top surgeons. Some of the Italian operations are known as the Picasso lift: You come out with one breast pointing north and the other southwest.

One evening, while discussing plastic surgery in Rome with Pitangui, the famous Brazilian surgeon, who is an old friend, I explained my point of view about motivation. I am honest, I said. I know I have had surgery done for myself. It cannot give you love. Why pretend we do it for men? It is a form of narcissism, perfectionism, or just plain healthy ego.

Pitangui replied, "Many of my cosmetic surgery patients are normal people who give their defect an abnormal importance. Suppose a man has a razor scar. If it reminds him of a bad background and of brothels, he wants it removed. If it came from a duel, he might be proud of it. A woman comes in with a big nose, but that is not the problem. She doesn't even know she has the nose. She's concerned with a spot on her leg, perhaps because it came when she couldn't do anything about it. It disturbs her because it reminds her of hard times."

Pitangui believes that to perform cosmetic surgery, one should have full training in reconstruction work. Many times, repairing a nose for cosmetic reasons results in knowledge that helps in a harelip or an abdominal operation, and vice versa. Even in functional surgery, there is an attempt to obtain an esthetic effect. His patients are evenly divided between those needing functional surgery and those wanting cosmetic surgery.

There are various cosmetic cases in which Pitangui refuses to intervene. One such case is a person emphasizing a minimal defect out of basic insecurity. Unless balance, possibly with the help of a psychiatrist, is found, the operation would solve nothing. There would be another defect the next day in a vain attempt to evade an insecurity that surgery cannot heal. Another case is the patient personally not disturbed by a defect but only following friendly advice. A third is when surgery is thought the solution to a husband's flirtation with another woman.

"The patients for cosmetic surgery that I have divide up roughly according to age: The youngest group comes for nose or acne and the oldest group for face-lifting. In between are the breasts and bellies."

The ideal time for women who are concerned with keeping their beauty is just after forty, when they are still well and there is the best chance of physical improvement. "I wish women wouldn't come to me when they are finished," he concluded.

I belong to the category of women who seek out the surgeon long before they are finished. I had

Pitangui do my eyes two years ago. They were all right, mind you, but they were not what they used to be. I prefer not to wait until something drastic has to be done. There is no sense trying to come out smooth as a baby when you go in looking like an old topographic map. Big, radical liftings scare me a little. Were they ever to drop, they might drop completely.

In the case of my eye operation, Pitangui suggested doing only the upper lid. This was because I showed no tendency toward bags under the eyes. Had I had incipient bags, the lower lid would have been done as well. The reason for having the upper lid lifted, even when it is not droopy or wrinkled, is that it opens up the eye—the wider, the smoother the space between eye and brow, the more the eye is set off. I was out of the clinic in twenty-four hours, returning three days later to have the stitches removed. Pitangui believes in getting you up and out as quickly as possible. I have the kind of skin that heals well. Within a week of the operation, nothing showed.

Another woman might recover even more quickly or take much longer. The vital issue is not recovery time but quality of the operation. You are only as good as your last plastic surgery. Once a poor job is done, it is much harder to repair it than to start from scratch. Cosmetic surgery need not be fabulously expensive, but it is nothing to save pennies on.

Surgery cannot work miracles. We have all met women who are furious because their lifts did not turn out as well as they had expected. Possibly, the results they wanted could not be achieved. When a face is badly furrowed, lifting can minimize the wrinkles and make them appear less deep, but it cannot eliminate them totally.

On the other hand, it is equally foolish to keep the plastic surgeon from achieving the greatest change possible. This is often the case when a woman is so petrified that people might find out she has had a lift, she insists that the operation be done in such a way that no one can see the difference. I remember the sad story of a London blepharoplasty (eye-lift) that was done to exactly that specification. After three weeks of dark glasses, the new woman returned to Rome and went to a beautician for candid advice on makeup and other improvements. The beautician innocently suggested an eye-lift. If I go, I tell a surgeon that I want very much to see the difference. Otherwise, why have it done?

Subterfuges in order to slip away for surgery are understandable enough: for example, saying you are going to your sister's place in the mountains where there is no telephone and going instead to a clinic for five days. Just be honest with yourself: You want to look better and you want everyone to notice it, whether or not they know why.

Subterfuges are rarer than they used to be because cosmetic survery has become a normal recourse for more and more people. In some cases, it can become a professional obligation like makeup for politicians and pundits on television. It is obvious you cannot be convincing about beauty and chic looking like the wrath. Right or wrong, almost any idea is more convincing when the person who conveys it does not look old and tired and down at the mouth.

A case in point is Gore Vidal, not because he

looks decrepit (on the contrary, he looks quite marvelous). But, in addition to writing, he frequently appears on television. "I wonder about eye-lifting," he says. "For normal life, I'd never consider it. Yet when you are on TV, every line shows. You get a bit depressed. On the other hand, there is no law that says I have to watch myself."

Again, I think it all comes down to whether your real image and your image of yourself are one and the same. Even without the pressure of public appearances, one can need the new lease on life that surgery helps to bring. The little old lady librarian explained that she saved her money to have her face lifted by a famous surgeon because "I have to live with myself, and I want to look well instead of all saggy."

In the beauty "establishment" of Rome, opinions vary on lifts as they do in any group. Marella Agnelli, who is very disciplined about keeping in top form, would not have surgery done for cosmetic reasons. She does not believe in attaching that much importance to her face. "Ultimately the fight against aging is lost," she says. "Unless your beauty has been truly exceptional, putting all your passion there can only make you neurotic."

Most women who go in for surgery pretend they have not, and I think not telling about it is like not telling your age. You might as well, because without the facts, the cynics' delight is to make you out to be more plastic and older than you are. One of the current jokes is that there is a midget running around Rome composed of what was cut off a prominent social figure. The dowager still pretends she is just as God made her.

Princess Virginia Ira von und zu Furstenberg,

THE
LOOK
AND HOW TO GET IT

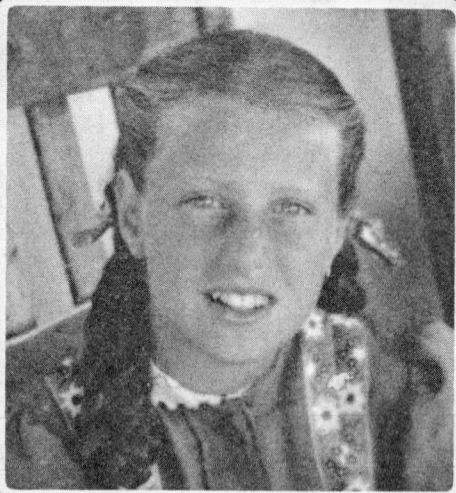

The author at twelve was all legs and big feet, thick at the waist and thick in the nose. She complained that her friends already had bosoms while she had only a chest.

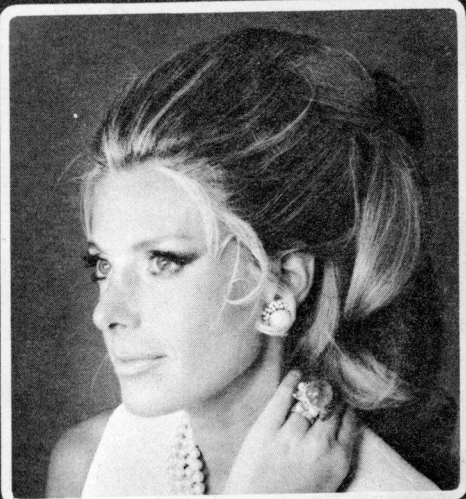

Today, the author believes in dazzle —
all the tricks and flourishes that can
make a woman glamorous.
—PHOTOGRAPH BY ELISABETTA CATALANO

Countess Consuelo Crespi, the author's sister-in-law, feels that working gives your life a sense of perspective. "If I hadn't worked, I would have been hysterical raising children." She has two children, Brando, twenty-one, and Pilar, nineteen.
—PHOTOGRAPH BY ELISABETTA CATALANO

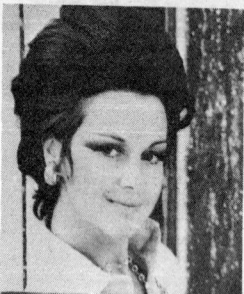

Veruschka, the cover girl, feels that a woman is most attractive when she acts her age.
—PHOTOGRAPH BY FRANCO RUBARTELLI

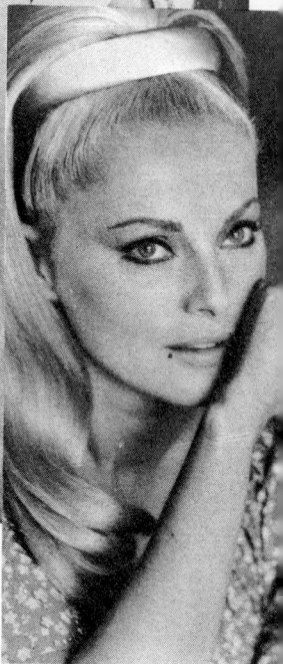

Virna Lisi is an expert with her hair and make-up as well. She should be — she's been experimenting and practicing since she was twelve.
—PHOTOGRAPH BY PIETRO PASCUTTINI

Sophia Loren, one of the world's
most beautiful and famous women.
—PHOTOGRAPH BY TAZIO SECCHIAROLI

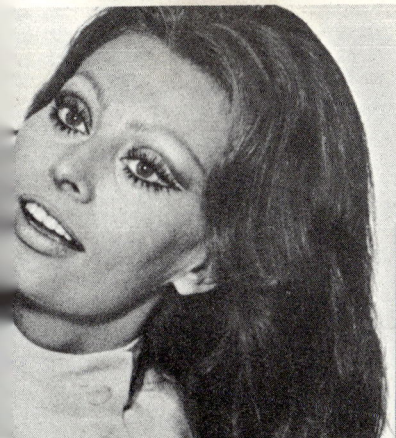

Princess Ira Von Furstenberg
is the picture of luscious
self-indulgence. Yet
her regimen is austere:
early to bed, early to rise,
no smoking, no drinking,
and two hours a day at the
gym when she is
not making a movie.
—PHOTOGRAPH BY
ELISABETTA CATALANO

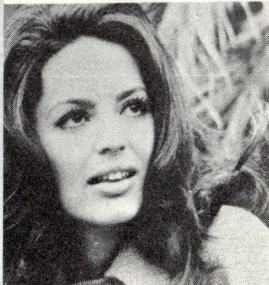

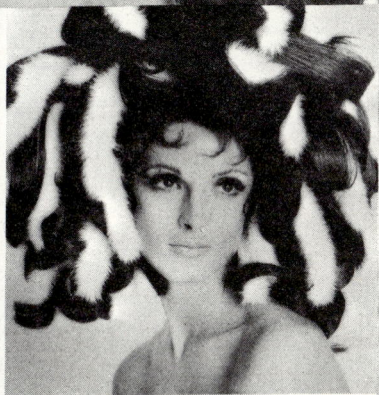

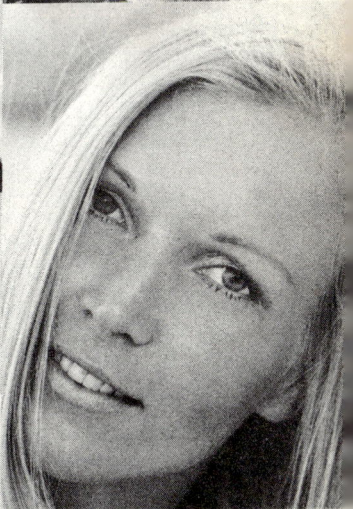

Mirella Haggiag, former cover girl,
is now Rome editor of
Italian Vogue. Her beauty philosophy
is simple:
"When you think food, you get fat."
—PHOTOGRAPH BY ELISABETTA CATALANO

Buxy Gancia, a former
Chanel model, is thirty;
although she is the mother
of two children, she
still has the body of an
adolescent. Few women
look better than she in a
sweater and pants.
—PHOTOGRAPH BY JEAN CLAUDE SAUER

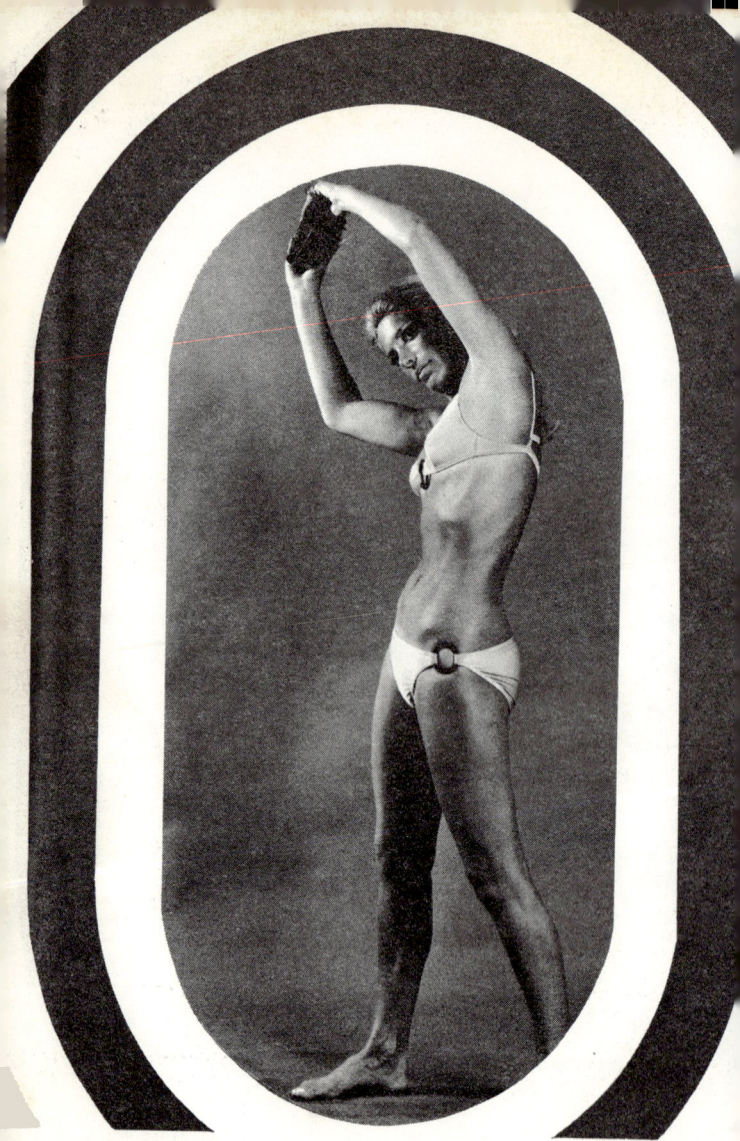

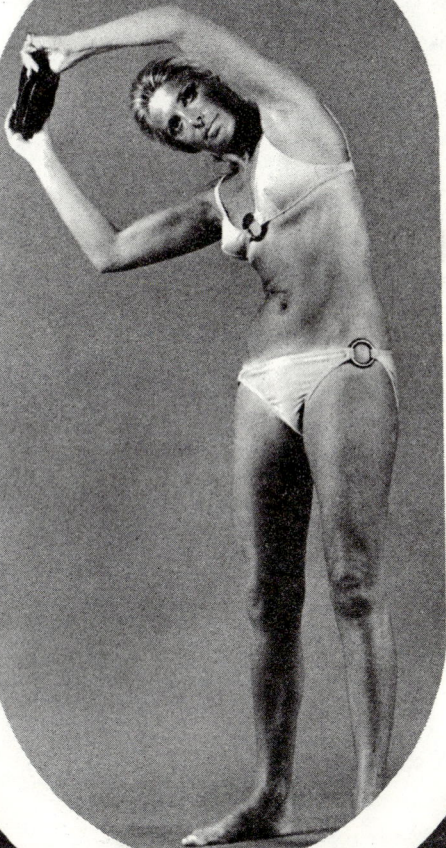

Windmill Tilt: Stand with legs apart, weights clasped in both hands with arms extended over your head. Lower both arms slowly to one side and slowly bring arms back to initial position. Exercise must be done **very** slowly to get maximum pull on waist and middle. Alternate sides, once to the left side, once to the right 10 times, work up to 15. **Marvelous for controlling the midriff and shrinking the waist.**

—PHOTOGRAPHS BY ALDANESI

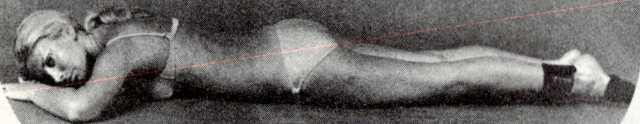

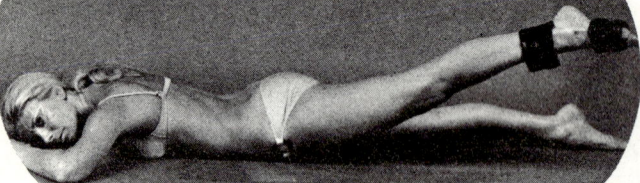

Extended Leg Kick: Stretch out prone, raise weighted leg upward and outward, keeping leg straight so that you feel a pull from the hip down. Lower leg slowly to the floor. Repeat 20 times with each leg, work up to 35 times. **Excellent for general leg toning.**

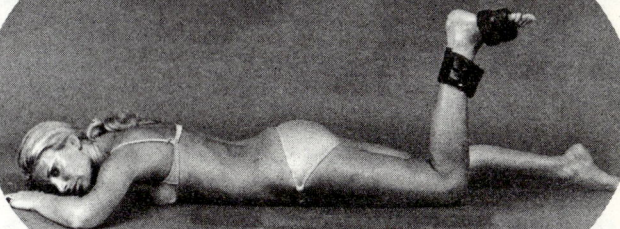

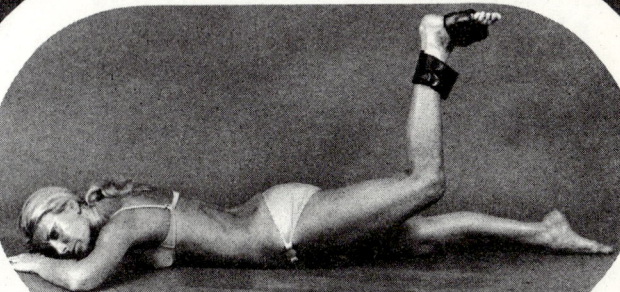

Bent Leg Pull: Stretch out prone, lift the lower half of weighted leg, bending the knee. Then, keeping the knee bent, lift the entire leg upward and outward. Repeat 20 times with each leg, work up to 35 times. **Good for tightening the front of the thigh.**

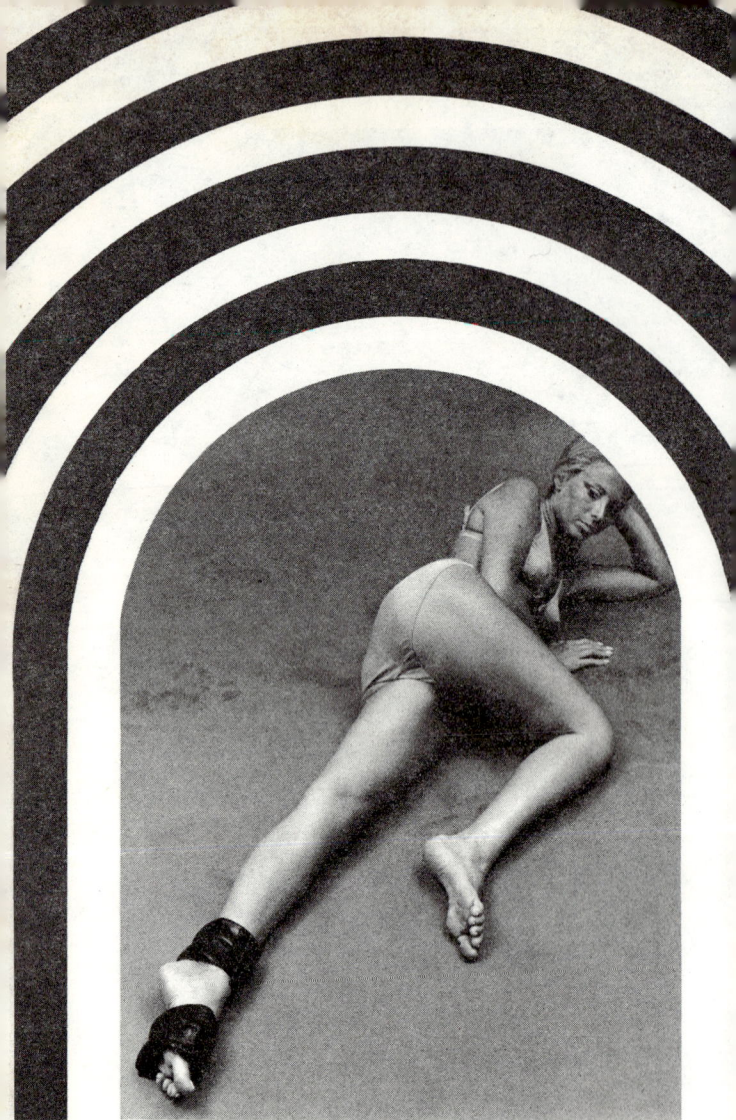

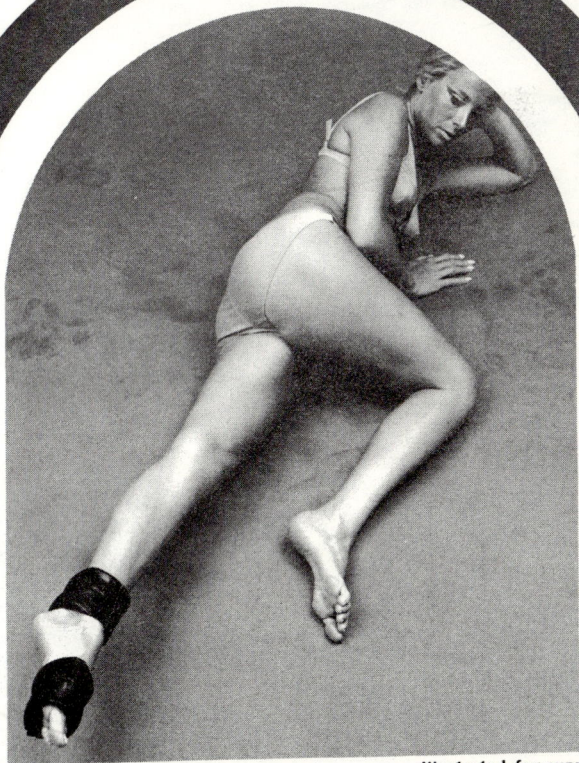

Inner Thigh Lift: Stretch out on side, using arms as illustrated for support. Bring top leg to the side, bending the knee. Lift bottom leg (weighted) and lower slowly. Repeat 20 times with each leg, work up to 30. **Tightens the muscles at the inside of the thigh.**

—PHOTOGRAPHS BY ALDANESI

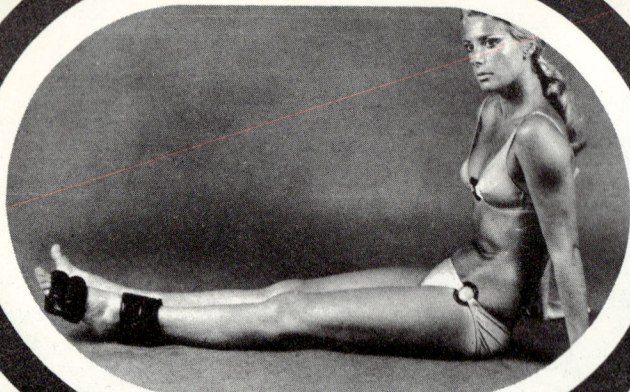

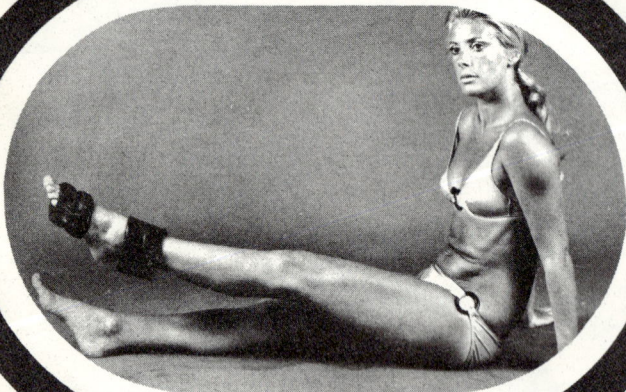

Extended Leg Stretch: Sit with arms at sides, hands pressing the floor, legs out straight. Lift leg with weights around ankle and instep upward and outward slowly. Lower slowly. Repeat 20 times. Change weights to other leg and repeat. **Trims the entire leg and tightens the buttocks.**

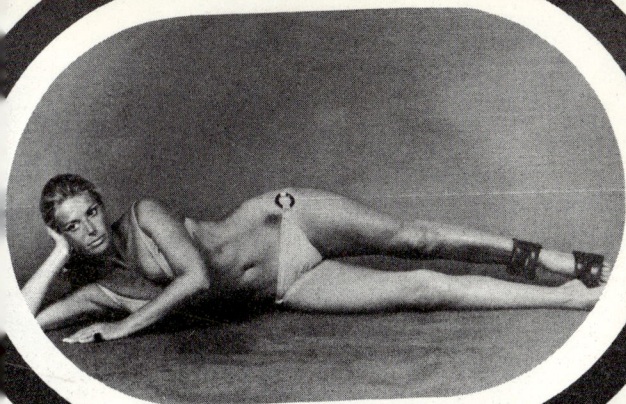

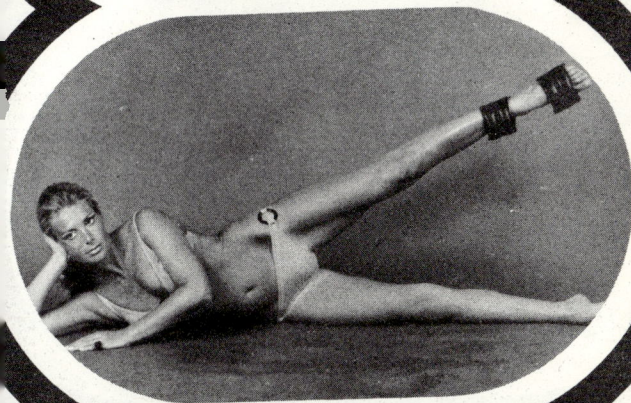

Outer Thigh Lift: Stretch out on side, using arms as illustrated for support. Lift weighted leg slowly and lower even more slowly. Repeat 20 times, then change weights to other leg, turn on other side, and repeat 20 times with other leg. **Reduces that bulge on the outside of the thigh.**

—PHOTOGRAPHS BY ALDANESI

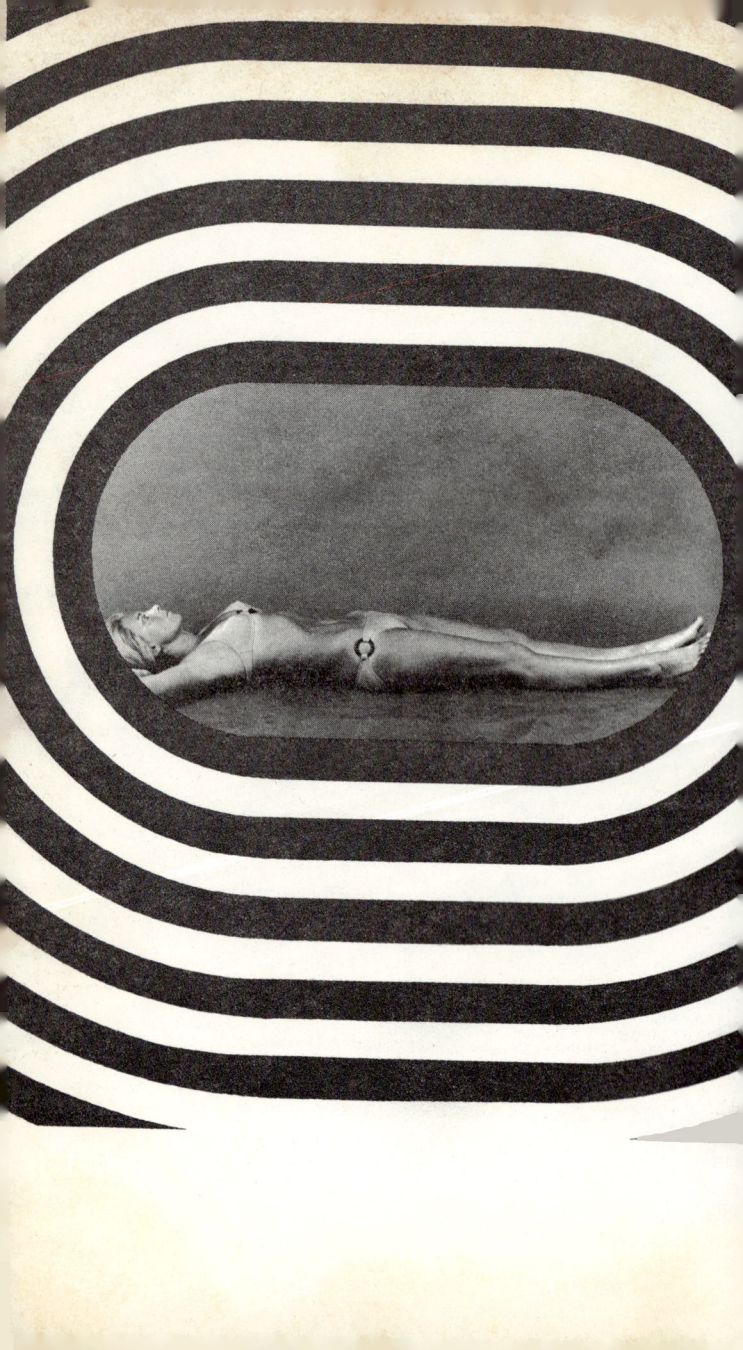

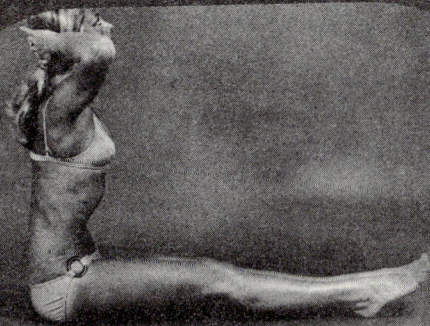

Abdominal Stretch: Stretch out flat on your back, with arms bent at the elbows, hands behind your head. Keeping the arms in the position shown, and your legs flat on the floor, slowly pull your body up to a sitting position and then slowly return to your initial position. Start with 20 times and work up to 30. **Flattens the tummy nicely.**

—PHOTOGRAPHS BY ALDANESI

Umbrella Exercise: Stand with legs apart, grasp umbrella (or stick) near the ends and hold at shoulder level. Tighten and relax grip as if trying to break umbrella. Repeat 10 times, work up to 15. Repeat the exercise holding umbrella near the center another 10 times, work up to 15. **Excellent for pectoral muscles — fills out that scrawny look.**

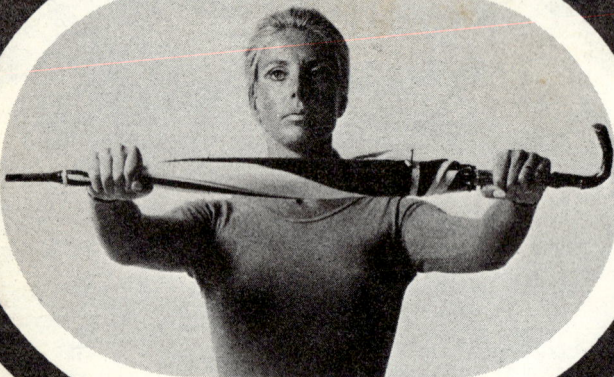

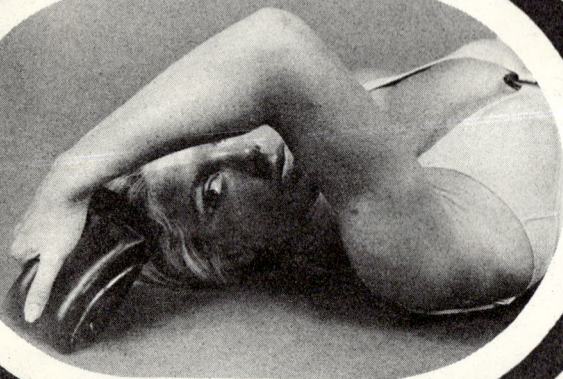

Applause Exercise: Stretch out on your back, holding weights in one hand with arm bent at elbow as shown. Keeping upper arm stiff, slowly raise and lower forearm. Repeat 5 times with each arm, work up to 10 times. **Tightens under side of upper arm (that flabby skin that quivers when you applaud).**

—PHOTOGRAPHS BY ALDANESI

who is thirty, is more candid about her lift. As an actress, she had it done for professional reasons. "I have a full face," she said. "It will be a big help when I'm forty, because it is the kind of face that stays up better. But the camera tends to broaden a face and make it look fat. Tightened at the sides, it's more photogenic."

Ira also says that instead of submitting to the torture of tapes to pull up the eyes, one might as well have them lifted surgically. She hated the tapes when they made her wear them for films and suspects that ultimately they stretch the skin and make it sag.

Talitha Getty, on the contrary, is still in the non-surgery ranks. She prefers to try and stay in shape as long as possible. Perhaps she will consider the idea of surgery later. Veruschka also says, "Maybe in ten to fifteen years," but is undecided. Rejuvenation and silicone shots worry her. As for lifting, if it is the way to change something you really hate, why not? She hopes that by the time she has to decide, lifting will be out of fashion. There will be some kind of pill instead.

"Perhaps if one starts early enough, does just a little, goes on for awhile . . ." she wonders. "Yet people who do all that lifting lose so much and look so stiff. There must be some other interest in life. If, when I'm forty to forty-five, I'm with a man who wants me to look twenty-five, he'll be the wrong man for me. It would be such a terrible struggle. There's such terror about getting old. In a way I really like women who show they have lived. My mother is still a beautiful woman and she has wrinkles. It's what comes out of the eyes that counts."

With her bone structure at age twenty-nine, the problem of losing her looks is unreal to Veruschka. Yet one of the most charming New York plastic surgeons, Thomas D. Rees, tells me that eyelid operations often are done in the late twenties and early thirties. In many women that is when the skin and fat bags around the eyes start to develop.

In Dr. Rees's experience, most face-lifting begins in the forties and continues from then on. (Mainly, this is true of women, but more and more men are becoming clients.)

The doctor explains that flat-chested girls have implants to increase the size of their breasts at any age, usually in their twenties. Reduction of big breasts is also done at any age, but most often in middle age or right after the childbearing period. Building up breasts, according to the surgeon, rarely affects lactation or sensitivity. Reducing them sometimes reduces sensitivity temporarily, and when they are huge, lactation must be interfered with. He finds that most women prefer loss of lactation to a heavy, pendulous bosom that makes it difficult for them to dress and causes grooves in their shoulders and aches in their backs and necks.

Dr. Rees does not entirely agree with me about the motivation for cosmetic surgery. I say a woman does it for herself and her mirror. If bags under the eyes and a few wrinkles stop anyone from having love or sex, they are not liable to have them after surgery either. The doctor protests: "Many times I have seen women who had bags under their eyes and a little sloppy loose skin around their jaws and necks become much more attractive physically after surgery, and also emotionally, because they gain confidence in themselves and then take more care of their hairdo, makeup, and so forth. In short, they become more attractive and do attract men, whereas before they did not. The surgery may not help their performance in bed, but it will certainly help them to get to bed."

I feel he is right—at least, in part. One of the reasons I have always tried to perfect the way I look is that I thought it would make me happier. Happiness for me does not exist without a man and love. But the drive for perfection in personal beauty, if not necessarily an end in itself, is still an inner drive, a compulsion, a self-imposed discipline that makes you wash that hair, watch that food, have that lift, get that sleep, take that walk —for your own self-respect.

Once I went to Dr. Rees for silicone injections. I have a long oval face, the kind that tends to get "smile lines." Fuller, tauter cheeks would smooth them out. I was given two tiny injections, one under each cheekbone. It was much like getting a shot at the dentist. It hurt, but only for a moment. The same evening I went out to dinner with friends. With less pronounced lines, my face appears more rested.

The rule with silicone is to be extremely careful in choosing the doctor, to make sure that the silicone is of the purest quality, and to have it injected only in minute quantities. In addition to Dr. Rees, I had very good results with dermatologist Dr. Michael Kalman's treatments in New York. Silicone injections should be done early so that the wrinkles are counteracted when they are just starting to form. It is also advisable to space the treatments, having a little done every three to four weeks rather than all at once if you are attacking more than one wrinkle. When the amounts injected are small, a subcutaneous growth can form around the silicone, holding it in permanent suspension. This gives the desired plumping effect and minimizes the risk of suddenly finding it all in your ears.

If I had one hundred beauty operations that did not show, that would be all right with me. It is the way you look that counts, not how you got that way. It only matters when an artifact looks phony, pops out or comes off at the wrong moment. He moves in for the first kiss, the false eyelash drops—romance dies.

I understand there is a Paris doctor who does eyelash implants. Next time I go to Paris, I intend to look into it. If they can be done properly, what a marvelous idea! One has them put in dark and just the right length. Then the days of messing with mascara would be over. You too must find it infuriating in the movies when you get the close-up of the star awakening—nobody has lashes like that when they first wake up. But the day may be coming.

6 Beauty from the Neck Down

No one in the world looks better in sweater and pants than former Chanel model Buxy Gancia as she runs, her long hair flying, down the lawn of her house near Lausanne. At thirty, after two children, she has the body of an adolescent. Buxy never bothers with gyms and massage. With her active outdoor life, she does not have to. She rides and golfs. When the weather is warm, she swims in the lake, and three months a year she skis at Gstaad and St. Moritz. Furthermore, she does a bit of yoga.

Confronted with Buxy, one accepts her superb form with grace. One can always think, "I'd have a great figure, too, if I lived her kind of life." But then you run up against the really maddening phenomenon: the woman who keeps a beautiful young body with almost no effort. Such creatures, fortunately for one's morale, are rare. I know of two. Former French *Vogue* editor Françoise de Langlade, now married to fashion designer Oscar de La Renta, does not exercise because it would make her too muscular. Ursula Andress needs little exercise for the same reason.

Would we were all so blessed! Most women, including myself, need a regular program of body care. When summer arrives, who has not had that "I don't dare to be seen in a bathing suit" feeling? It is bad enough to be all white the first day on the beach without uncovering fat as well.

"Beauty has a larger dimension than it used to," says designer Emilio Pucci. "Thirty years ago, the body didn't matter so much. Now it does. We live a nuder life. A person of quality," he insists, "simply cannot allow himself to have a big stomach any more than he would live in a disorderly, messy house."

An American hairdresser once scoffed, as I heard through the grapevine, "Oh, of course, Luciana Pignatelli is always in shape. She has had everything lifted, even her bottom." I may have had problems with my bottom, but what I do about it is exercise and massage.

You may be made of sturdier stuff. I find I have to exercise regularly. If I stop, in a few months the body begins to go. It has always been that way. When I was eighteen, I rode a lot in Villa Borghese. As soon as I no longer had the time and gave up daily riding, the muscle dissolved. Living in Rome, I slip off to the beach at weekends five months of the year. And I do not laze through the other seven, much as I would like to.

As with eating, so with exercise: Every woman has to find her own equilibrium. Apart from sports, if you practice them, massage may be enough for you. It hardly ever is. In my experience, massage without exercise does nothing.

Depending on temperament, the ideal year-round answer may be hatha-yoga, "the path of physical perfection." It is not the answer for the man who wants to be a paragon of muscle power, nor for the woman with a figure problem who wants to spot reduce or achieve specific measurements. In its physical aspect, what hatha-yoga does do is balance the body, keep it in line and, through correct breathing, increase endurance. Often it reshapes the body, but essentially it restores it or keeps it at peak. The other great enhancement that comes with yoga is youthful suppleness. A body that cannot move and bend freely, no matter how slender and pampered, no longer looks young. Few defects give away age quicker than rigidity.

"There is no sense having your face lifted," Grant Muradoff, my Rome yogi, says, "when you're wobbling on your feet or walking like a duck with a mink coat." And going beyond appearance, as yogis are prone to do, Muradoff adds, "I remember watching one of those women with Blanche de Vries, my teacher. 'For God's sake,' she exclaimed, 'what can she do in bed?' "

Needless to say, yoga's special appeal is to people who believe in the body beautiful as a stepping-stone to mental and physical harmony. It is particularly effective with people who do not fear intensity, but suffer instead from tension, which can age you rather badly. Yoga movements, unlike calisthenics, are never brisk or fatiguing. They are slow and stretchy, based on complementary opposites: *ha* ("sun") and *tha* ("moon"), push and pull, up and down, left and right, effort and release. It is this constant balancing that shows up both in body form and in new psychic energy.

Much as I appreciate yoga, my personal choice is to work out in a gym only because I do not have time for both. And when one must choose, the only criterion is to do whatever works best for you.

By temperament, I happen to be very beauty-conscious, also very lazy. There are people, and I

hope you are one of them, who have never lost
their childhood delight in the body's infinite re-
sources and therefore adore expending themselves.
I do it out of necessity and self-discipline. To see
the body degenerate, no matter how little, disturbs
me profoundly. I think it disturbs most women.
While I know that yoga is beneficial in the long
run, I go to the gym because it is the most convincing antidote to laziness. It gives me the
quicker, tangible results I must have to get me to
exercise.

Having done gym work for years, I have even
evolved a series of basic movements that can be
done at home. The movements are illustrated at
the end of this chapter, and the only equipment
required is weighted circlets. Mine happen to be
"Voight," but Faye Dunaway used to tie bags of
sand on her waist, wrists, and ankles to serve the
same purpose. Instead of doing an exercise an un-
bearably boring one hundred times, with weights
thirty times is enough. Before I discovered ready-
mades, I had bullets sewn up into wearable
weights. To my mind, more complicated apparatus
is useless. Machines always wind up in a closet as
soon as their initial fascination wanes. Furthermore, they cannot be packed in a suitcase, and
with exercise, do-it-yourself is an expedient for
when you cannot have an expert to guide you. Do-
it-yourself is the traveler's boon.

"I have a machine I haven't used for months because it needs a battery," Veruschka admits. "It's
really too much trouble to take all that stuff out
and put it on. Supposedly you can lie down and
read while it makes your muscles jump. But really

you can't, and you're aware that all that twitching is rather grotesque."

"If I have an appointment to exercise with someone, I go," says Mirella Haggiag. "If it's just an appointment with myself or a machine, I put it off."

Most of us put it off. When we are settled at home, there are too many distractions. The phone rings; children need attention; the dog comes in; the maid has a question; the plumber arrives. All of them are excellent excuses. And not being experts, we justly wonder after awhile whether we are doing the best movements in the best possible way. Like Mirella, I find that going to a professional is more businesslike and efficient. One gets organized, finds the time, and goes, perhaps gleaning the bonus of feeling extra virtuous because one has fought a traffic jam to get there.

The only sort of exercise that is forever successful at home is the kind that appeals to the imagination. For example, Talitha Getty lives at the top of an old palazzo. The three flights of impressive entrance stairs were designed so that horses could be driven up them. They are not just any old dull stairway. Talitha enjoys walking up them and easily adds special exercise for good measure. She does the stairs two steps at a time on tiptoe.

There is also one other circumstance in most women's lives when home exercise and massage are of great value. I refer to pregnancy and postnatal care. During pregnancy, as the belly ripens and rounds, it is folly not to gently massage it with cream or oil. Why have stretch marks when often they can be avoided? Personally, I massaged morning and evening or whenever the opportunity presented itself, with oil. There are many alternatives, from flour and simple coconut butter to exotic preparations, but none work if they just sit there in the medicine cabinet.

Here I would add another word to the wise from Talitha. During pregnancy, many women also become heavier in the upper thighs. If so, massage them with cream as well, or they too may bear post-pregnancy marks. On the other hand, Talitha was advised, erroneously as she discovered, to wear a maternity girdle. "It was my first baby," she said, "and a girdle was totally unnecessary. If you wear one, it takes you much longer to get back into shape."

After pregnancy, swimming is excellent for regaining one's figure. But for a variety of reasons, not everyone prefers or arranges to have late-spring babies. One young Finnish beauty whose first Roman baby hardly affected her at all found she did not spring back into shape after the second. She coped by buying a bicycle and cycling up a storm for several months.

The classic home remedies are abdominal exercises that can be done stretched out on floor or bed. The first is simply a form of deep breathing, first on the back and then on the sides. During prolonged exhaling, one makes a special effort to suck in the abdominals before pushing them out for inhalation. The others are pull-ups in addition to what both Sophia Loren and Talitha describe as the "up and downs." This means lying on the back and swinging up the legs and lowering them as slowly as possibly. The umbrella-breaking exercise, shown at the end of this chapter, helps strengthen the pectoral muscles, which also need special attention at this time.

But, when well-organized at home and happily nonpregnant—after two children that is over with, I think—it is more effective and quite sufficient to exercise out of the house. In Rome, my favorite physical education expert is Professor Enzo Sbarra. Whatever good form I attain, I owe to him, and so do most of the beautiful people in Rome. The professor, who combines exercise with massage, is the Pininfarina of the female body. He takes a woman who looks like a dump truck, or a matron who is fast becoming a tank, and turns her into a Ferrari.

"I can't eliminate all bad design," he protests. "First I work on contour and attack the obvious defects to give a woman confidence in the results. Then I try to correct the others, because for me health and esthetics are linked."

Surely every big city has at least one good gym. The trick is to find it, go to the best instructor, and take private rather than group lessons. I can talk about Sbarra because I have seen what he has done to women's thick ankles; badly shaped legs; pear, apple, and floating island shapes. His clients may not come out with the body of Raquel Welch, but they do emerge with their own personal structure perfected. To my mind, taking standardized group lessons is a waste of time unless all you need is maintenance therapy. If you have particular problems, and most women who go to a gym do or they would not bother, then you need personal attention.

Sbarra's great strength is that he is also concerned with insides and attitudes. A good gym instructor is not necessarily a psychiatrist, but if he ignores mental hygiene, it limits his effectiveness. To cite a very simple example: Consuelo Crespi sent her daughter Pilar to Sbarra when she was eighteen. Pilar did not have a figure problem. She was sent to acquire preventive habits—things like not drinking ten Cokes a day and not always sitting with her legs crossed. (You tend to cross your legs with the same one always on top. In the long run, the inner thigh of the under leg gets flabby as a result.)

Exercising, ideally, is part of a disciplined way of life that carries over from one session to another. If a gym instructor never asks about how you sleep, what you eat, what pills you take, and whether you have any deficiencies, he is not very serious about his work.

Some of the most valuable tips I learned from Sbarra concern the hygienic considerations of dress and hairstyle. He says that hairstyles and clothing that are constricting must be avoided for regular use. Obviously, this means tight wigs, clamped-in hairpieces, or tight belts. But girdles also are anathema—that was the first thing he made me throw out. You must work at developing the muscles instead.

With a small bosom, exercise and toning with blasts of cold water do more for you than a bra. I hardly ever wear one now. And although exercising the pectorals does not enlarge the bosom, it fills out that scrawny, bony look.

For women whose larger breasts need the support of a bra, Sbarra warns against wearing the same style all the time. If possible, they should change bras at least once a day. Even if you prefer one style because it is the most comfortable and flattering, it should be alternated with another design. Wearing one style only means constant constriction in the same places.

Sbarra also detests stockings because of all the rig you have to wear to keep them up. Tights or panty-hose are a far more sensible solution. As for tight shoes or heels high enough to throw off posture, no one who goes to the professor wears them for long.

When I weigh in at 127 pounds (for a 5' 7" frame), Sbarra only has me exercise, mostly without weights. He reserves the weights, in my case, for muscles that tend to go slack because they are never used in my sort of life. Were I scurrying up trees to harvest coconuts and dates, no doubt my thigh muscles would not need weights.

When I go to 130 pounds, it is back to the heat lamps and massage as well as exercise. As most women past their first youth have discovered, extra pounds do not necessarily take the form of solid plumpness. This might not be so objectionable. Instead this extra fat shows up as cellulite.

Cellulite is that most unattractive fat that looks like orange rind when squeezed. It tends to form on hips or thighs, sides of the knees, upper arms, or back of the neck. There are infinite conflicting theories about cellulite's cause and cure. Doctors object to the term as inaccurate. But when they see the "orange rind" syndrome, they recognize it as a pathological state and call it cellulite for lack of a better term. Rome's Dr. Alberto Lodispoto defines it as a biochemical alteration of the basic connective tissue substance. He, for one, is sure there is no one cause. That would be too easy. Sometimes it is linked to obesity, but often it shows up in people who are thin or of normal weight for their size.

He also claims it is not a sickness in itself, but a symptom, like fever or a headache, of other disorders that must be diagnosed. The origin may be functional, like flat feet that throw the spinal column out of line; it may be a metabolic disorder or an endocrine dysfunction. He suspects that when more doctors begin to look into it seriously, instead of shrugging it off as a cosmetic problem, there will be pills or shots to cure it.

For the moment, massage, if not the definitive cure, still appears to be the best palliative. Again, there is disagreement on the type of massage most suitable for cellulite. Dr. Lodispoto is of the opinion that in the initial phase only the lightest massage is correct. He compares it to treating someone who has a fracture. In the beginning one must go easy but, as the fracture mends, deeper massage aids articulation and mobility. If you emerge from your first massage treatments with black and blue marks, the doctor says, "Shoot the masseur."

I can only speak from my experience. In addition to exercise, Sbarra uses heat lamps to treat the area afflicted by cellulite, then uses both machine and manual massage that is as thorough as one can take. His theory is that cellulite stops capillary circulation. Even with strong massage, if cellulite has really set in, the area invaded does not at first respond by getting pink. The blood has to be brought back into the afflicted area. He also recommends slapping the area alternately with hot and cold sponges or washcloths at home between treatments. My mirror tells me that Sbarra's system works. If I do nothing for several months, the cellulite returns. As long as I keep after it, it disappears.

I, personally, am so fiercely anticellulite that I have supplemented Sbarra not only with a masseur who comes to the house, but also with experiments in Dr. Kurt Ekman's diacutaneous fibrolysis. The latter is used to combat various types of pathological fibrous formation in soft tissue such as chronic rheumatism and post-fracture femoral inflammations. Dr. Ekman, who now lives and works in Rome, has published his findings in medical journals, but the technique is far from becoming a household word.

According to Ekman, manual manipulation can only penetrate so far. He has devised a series of small hooked instruments that he uses to reach deeper and loosen fibrous adhesions. Were he not such a gentle person, the tall, austere, thin-faced doctor with his hooked instruments in hand would be a formidable sight.

When I had no cellulite—and I am not exactly afflicted by masses of it—his explorations did not hurt. Where there were cellulite adhesions, it did in the beginning. But when the doctor had loosened them up, my masseur found it much easier to work because the cellulite was detached. Ekman warned me that I risked getting small broken veins from diacutaneous fibrolysis. If you are in great pain from some traumatic fibrous formation, then obviously relief is worth a few little vein marks on the skin. There is no sense getting them just to speed up removal of cellulite. But I would risk trying any possible beauty cure, and all I noticed were somewhat bruised-looking scratch marks that disappeared in a day or two.

Massage alone rarely corrects any defect, including cellulite. It encourages too passive an attitude, whereas you have to use muscles and work at keeping in form. Yet as long as they do not delude themselves that it gives them effortless beauty, I understand people who adore to be slowly, gently, soothingly massaged. All the kinks and contrariness of the day are pulled out. The tensions disappear. Depending on how it is done, massage either stimulates or tranquilizes—and far better, in the long run, than any pill.

Veruschka says that someday, when she is very rich, she would love to employ a personal masseur who would travel with her. "I get very tense," she explains, "and one's own masseur is the ultimate luxury."

"If I could be massaged before going to sleep, it would be fantastic," echoes Consuelo Crespi. "I just don't have the time."

Virna Lisi would settle for someone at her beck and call only to massage her feet. "I'd have it done over and over again," she says.

Talitha Getty, when not traveling, tries to have a masseur come to the house every other day. "I'm sure it makes a difference," she claims. "Linda Christian has a girl's body and she is a fiend for massage."

Nor is it only women who purr under skillful hands. Gianni Agnelli, the activist of all activists, tries to fit a thorough massage into his tight schedule, at least in the winter when he flies up for fast weekends at St. Moritz. I suppose it may be that the richer you are, the less you can relax, and what induces relaxation becomes vital. An hour, a half hour with a good masseur, and the batteries are recharged.

"I swim and ski and I have a very strong nervous system," Emilio Pucci says, "but when I'm tired, there is nothing like a half-hour massage. It is my drug. In Rome, I have two Filipino girls who come to the house. I would never be massaged by a man —I'd find it distasteful. One of the reasons why massage works is that it's erotic," he continues. "Don't misunderstand me, I am far from pretending that massage is sex or a substitute for it. But anything so physical, so involved with the sense of touch, has an erotic component that is revitalizing."

The most fantastic massage I ever had was in London. The method was aromatotherapy, and I wish I could have it done every week. This technique, based on absorption through the skin of essential oils, perfumes and aromatics, was launched by the late Marguerite Maury in her Chelsea clinic.

There are various aromatotherapists in London now, some of whom have special treatments for cellulite. I did not go for anything special. I went just for a basic massage to Dr. Richard Simpson, osteopath and former assistant to Madame Maury. First he did a blood test, then gave me a pressure-massage on back, decolleté, neck and face with the combination of essences he thought most suitable. He did not give me the formula, and each client's is different. Lemon grass might be included, or rose (thought to influence female sex organs), neroli from orange blossoms, patchouli, lavender or pepper (good for muscle atonia), etc.

The massage starts on the back. The doctor found so many knots, he asked if I had been in an accident. I had not; it was just accumulated tension. There is something both sacred and wildly luxurious in the idea of being anointed. Whether it was the fragrance, the massage, or, as practitioners claim, the combination of both, the effect was magic. You come out of aromatotherapy feeling magnificent.

(I also tried one of the doctor's beauty products, a moisturizer based on ginseng. Natural cosmetics now are in fashion. At that time, they were rare.)

Next to massage, one of the great body-beautiful pleasures is bathing. How nice, that in our culture, cleanliness is close to godliness. That way its doubtless erotic component passes as pristine virtue. When I moved into my new apartment, the first room I really thought out was the bathroom. Along with proper lighting for makeup, I had the floor and the walls carpeted and, while I was at it, the ceiling as well. With everything else in shining porcelain and stainless steel, the effect is rather like a fur-lined lab.

Bathroom carpeting for me is a must because I hate the alternatives of scampering into slippers or gingerly toeing the cold tile floor. But if you like the terrace effect of tile floors and plants, by all means have them. Candy stripes, paneling, rococo, rural primitives, Louis XIV with *chaise percée*— whatever makes you feel like indulging yourself is right. And if landlord basic suffices, stick to it and spend the money elsewhere.

Everyone must find their own cleansing rites. For some it is a luscious long bath. On the other hand, the last thing a woman with low blood pressure needs is soaking in hot water. It exhausts her. And even hot baths should never contain water higher than pelvic level. That is another tip I owe to my gym instructor—the part of the body underwater and the part above should be kept in blance. Above all, the bosom must never soak in the tub. Hot water only drags it down, and no woman wants that.

If you can stand them, alternate hot and cold showers tone the body. If that is too rigorous (I happen to loathe showering), after a warm bath, aim a good blast of cold water on bosom and thighs. They need it.

Consuelo Crespi does exercises after her evening bath because she is more relaxed then. Virna Lisi cannot resist those divine Floris bath oils; nor can Mirella Haggiag, who has a passion for cleanliness. Mirella has a shower in the morning and an hour-long bath every evening. She is embarrassed to think how much she spends at Floris on salts, perfumes, oils, water-softeners, and after-bath creams. Except for Saturday, the biggest bath day of the week, she substitutes oils for soap, which dries out her skin. In the winter, after her bath, she smoothes in baby oil to keep the skin supple. Another of her tricks is to put her makeup on before getting in the tub. Doing it that way "sets" the makeup.

As for the bath/shower controversy, it is not a male-vigor/female-languor thing at all. It is a question of temperament and physical need and should be respected as such. With men as with women, there are those who like to be stimulated and those who like to be soothed.

Nino Cerruti, handsome textile tycoon and fashion designer, is a long-distance commuter, spending half the week in Paris, half near Milan. He unwinds in the tub. When nervous—and what man in a highly unstable, competitive business is not—

he often takes two baths a day. The baths are tepid, and after them he likes a good brushing. If there is no brush around, rough treatment with a towel will do. And a beautiful girl to scratch his back is heaven.

Emilio Pucci believes that a foamy, good-smelling bath gives him strength when he is tired. He became interested in bath products while traveling and has now added them to his multifaceted collection. "There are no cities where the water smells good," he says. "You turn on your bath and the smell is awful. Yet breathing in something pleasant is very important while relaxing in the tub. It restores you."

Rudi Crespi agrees, pours bath oil into the water and soaks in the tub before going out for the evening. All the tensions of the day dissolve. And while lingering in the warm water, he sips an ice-cold vodka and tonic for contrast.

Buxy Gancia, on the other hand, is a shower person. She starts her day with a cold shower at 8 A.M. This would shatter me, but she thrives on it. Then she brushes with a rough brush, puts on body oil, and is ready for breakfast with the children. Gianni Agnelli is another who believes in a bracing start to the day—a cold shower, a few minutes exercise, and the metabolism is churning.

I am most decidedly a bath person—I love the slow, soothing effect. The number of daily baths depends on where I am. In Rome, a good evening bath is enough. In dirtier, more industrialized cities, twice a day is too little, but one does what one can.

Strangely enough, I am not attracted by thermal cures. I have tried the mud baths at Ischia (you sit in the hot mineral water and can almost see the blemishes vanish). But much as I believe in their regenerative results, I do not really enjoy them. One friend who tried the spas reported that, as a side effect, soaking in all the water makes you get pregnant even with a diaphragm. The establishments disclaim such surprise cures.

Bathing at home in ordinary water, which I prefer, is a busy as well as a relaxing moment. At change of season, and particularly after summer, I use a sturdy brush upwards on the skin against the grain to slough off dry cells and old tan. (It is a good idea during pregnancy, too.) Every two weeks, while in the tub, I give my back a good scrub with a loofah, a wet, soapy strip of vegetable sponge. Also, I alternate bath oil with a good slather of moisturizing lotion after I have toweled.

That is basic routine. Then, depending on need, come the variations, most of which I learned from Rome's leading chiropodist, Enzo d'Angiolillo. Enzo has done everyone's feet that matter—except, he regrets, Greta Garbo's. Even more to the point, he takes care of the two local soccer teams. As with masseurs, so with foot men: If they deal with athletes, they have to know what they're doing.

For cellulite, Enzo recommends one tablespoon of iodized alcohol in tepid bath water. As a nourisher for legs and feet, he says the only answer to dry, scaly skin is drugstore lanolin. For rheumatic aches and pains, he would add one tablespoon of Solvay soda per half-full tub of water. In the summer, the best (and cheapest) friction lotion for feet, legs, and body is 100 grams of camphorized alcohol, 1 gram of menthol, and 5 grams of lanolin oil. The blend, which reactivates circulation, is a quick pick-me-up.

Enzo believes in "non-soap" soap rather than regular soap for the body. This is particularly vital when feet present a perspiration problem. Sweat glands are acid, and putting a normally alkaline soap on them only burns. If the perspiration is nervous, bathing with water and vinegar helps. Pregnant women often find their feet perspire, but so do many men. Rather than plain talcum powder, which closes the pores and dries the skin, mentholated or camphorized talcum is in order. So is lanolin oil or the European "Fissan" powder.

Women with trim, smooth, attractive bodies are young women—mentally as well as physically. When your body is toned and gleaming, you feel better and healthier, and when you feel well you want to try new and exciting things. It is your enthusiasm that keeps you young, and (to come full circle) it is your zest for living that makes you take the time to look even better.

7 *Putting a Total Look Together*

When I stepped out of the elevator in a Houston office building last winter, a man stopped and stared. "Honey," he drawled, "you sure don't look Texan." I take this as proof that there really is a contemporary Italian look. Just after the war it was bosom and bottom and pointed shoes with spike heels. Now, it is just as easy to spot, but harder to define: a way with accessories, a good head of hair, a straight nose, a well-defined eye, a sense of sustaining bone under the surface. There is an open quality to the Italian face, a gaze that says, "I am ready to enjoy whatever falls into the net."

But faces are tricky; some of the best Italian looks now seem more for export than for native soil. They have taken on a cosmopolitan quality. Likewise, some of the most strongly Italian characteristics suddenly appear in the most unlikely places. Years ago, *Life* had a cover of a helmeted U.S. serviceman who was not of Italian origin. Yet he was pure Piero della Francesca, right off the church wall in Arezzo. And the living Botticellis in Italy in recent seasons have been English hippie girls.

For me, what is indefinable in the Italian look is more a style or attitude than any particular set of features. A relaxed open-air life is the basis of Roman beauty, but along with it goes careful attention to the sophisticated finishing touches. It is not so much clothes that make the Italian—the clothes can come from anywhere—it is a way of putting clothes, makeup, and hair together.

When I stepped off the elevator in Houston, along with Italian bag and shoes I was wearing an English dress, Kenny Lane and Bulgari jewels, and French panty-hose. Doubtless my hairstyle was "made in Italy" and so was my makeup, although the technique for the application of the latter may have been suggested by a Belgian specialist. Put them all together, they still spell R-O-M-A-N.

Whatever the components, I meant the effect to be as appealing as possible. Style for most Italian beauties, certainly for me, means all the glamour one can muster. On the one hand, we shun the extremes of hard chic or kinky disarray; on the other, we are not about to hide our looks. Generally, an Italian woman's innate fear of appearing ridiculous keeps her from diving off fashion's deep end. (I would even prefer that dive to the cult of understatement, which has always struck me as a waste of good spirit.)

The modern Roman beauty, in particular, never adheres long to the notion that a woman either looks like a lady or looks like she has a good time. Why should chic and knowledgeable beauty in any way detract from manners and decency? If one has manners and decency, they resist the most dire of circumstances and cannot suffer from one's looking as smashing, rather than as conservatively safe, as possible.

I adore to ride, for example, but I fail to see why certain society ladies in the horsy set should look so leathery and weather-beaten when the horses they ride are so well-groomed. I do not see why on a glorious night with the moon sailing high and jasmine on the terrace one should choose to appear in a little underplayed number that is already a bore at breakfast. (And probably a $900 bore at that—a strange sort of inverted snobbery.) Rather, be Italian! Wear something soft, seductive and, possibly, conspicuous.

Which is not to say that Roman beauties do not understand casual chic. On hot summer days, their look of simplicity is unbeatable. Although not every big city can turn into a baroque beach town when the barometer soars, the bare-legged, tanned approach of Rome is a style that both flatters the woman and respects the Fahrenheit. A slip of a dress, designed not to crumple, an amusing jewel, good sandals, and you are off for the day. Hair tied back with a scarf, no foundation, and never a speck of powder.

During the July round of fashion collections, the fashion editors always delight in coming to Rome. The schedule is as grueling as in other collection cities, but here, at least, they can abandon their gloves, closed shoes, and stockings with glee. When summer comes to Italy, you are supposed to look like summer. It makes sense and has developed into a supremely radiant style.

But as you might suspect, glamour, whether romantic, casual, or exotic, needs a good backbone to sustain it. The backbone in this case is organization down to the last detail. Fashion magazines all over the world continue to insist on the importance of a total look. A dress no longer matters. Whether it is bargain boutique or bargain basement, a simple dress worn with the right accessories and hairstyle can be more chic than a designer original with the wrong additions. (To be honest, if you complete an original with flair it usually beats the economy number.) The point is still the overall effect, not just the dress. There will always be a select group of women to maintain the haute couture, but most of us balk at spending so much money on clothes and prefer to invest in something that lasts more than a season.

Accessories have always been the heart of the Italian look and are now important everywhere. I can always spot an Italian beauty by her shoes, bag, and scarf; they are infallibly right in themselves and for what she is wearing. Her choices reflect an artisan tradition and a familiarity with the well-designed, well-made object. They also imply an enjoyment in searching out the perfect ring for one's hand and one's costume, the perfect proportion of a heel to a skirt of a certain cut and length.

Surely, this attention to every last detail in the overall effect stems in part from the competitiveness of Italian females. No flaw escapes them. An American woman will greet you by saying you look divine, but an Italian woman never pays you a compliment. If she goes so far as to say you look well, that is the day you are absolutely stunning.

Chic women anywhere know how to pull a look together; I think the Italian has an easier time because the components are less standardized—designers and craftsmen will alter a sample to a specific need if you insist and have patience. Even if you buy elsewhere and prefer ready-mades, the rule is to think in terms of what each item can be worn with. This becomes such a habit after awhile that sudden impulse buying is automatically integrated into the general wardrobe scheme. You simply do not buy that marvelous little thing that catches your eye in a shop window, unless it relates. You know that otherwise it will only stay in the closet or lead to a whole new rush of buying to justify the first impulse purchase.

The days of letting one designer think for you are over. There is no longer a fashion center that can dictate. You have to think out your own style, your own brand of glamour. Almost anything goes, as long as it goes together with you.

Beauties based in Rome, like their counterparts everywhere, travel so much that to integrate their scattered fashion gleanings they have to keep the overall plan in their heads. They may do the basic outline in Rome, then fill it not only in New York, London, or Paris, but more than likely in Bangkok, Lima, San Francisco, Morocco, Israel, Mexico, or Greece as well.

Talitha Getty loves to buy things in London to wear in Rome and vice versa. (She finds the amusing English clothes are often badly made, but a designer label is not the guarantee of workmanship it used to be.) Talitha's real sport, however, is riding the crest of the mania for costume, fantasy, and folklore. Why worry about coordinating clothes and accessories for evening when you acquire a far more extravagant total look in souks and bazaars?

From her travels in North Africa and the Middle East, Talitha has scads of caftans and Saudi Arabian robes, adores their intricate embroideries. To simplify her moving about, she leaves most of the North Africana in her Marrakesh house so she can travel light when Africa-bound. Oriental jewelry, a caftan, shoulder-length hair, kohl on the eyes to bring them out and play the inverted triangle of brow and cheekbones—the Talitha picture is complete. (In Marrakesh, before being donned, the caftan may have been hung over an engraved brass brazier in which wet sandalwood was tossed to smolder on the charcoal. It gives the caftan a marvelous smell.)

Last year, Talitha spent four months in the East and splurged on fabrics from Thailand, Laos, Indonesia, and Malaysia. One of them, a painting on cloth, was meant to be a wall hanging. "I hang it on me," she says. "It's like wearing the Balinese Bible. I'm going to do a room like that, too, in our new London house."

You may object that you do not have access to Eastern sources. The attitude is the point. If one loves costume, sources are infinite. The folklore trend started with imaginative girls who either were antiestablishment or could not afford establishment prices. Rather than envy and scrimp, they created a livelier style of their own, raiding thrift shops, attic trunks, and flea markets. Personally, I have my reservations on the folklore trend—more about that later.

Veruschka, who travels constantly as a model, seizes on traditional costume as a way to evolve a highly personal Veruschka look. For instance, she takes a Colombian *juana* or poncho and wears it with boots and ribbed tights and top. Instead of a mini, she adds a wide belt of tiger skin or leather. That was her look at the Valentino collection in which he launched the midi. Veruschka knew perfectly well what he was going to show. She showed her style instead. Tomorrow her style may change, but it will always be Veruschka.

"I prefer *juanas* because for me coats are finished," she explains. "All those seams and buttons are too complicated. I prefer the feeling of just having pieces of cloth around me. I'm no good at sewing. If I could just buy materials and cut something to cover me when I go out, that would be marvelous. I only like clothes that can be worn different ways so you don't get fed up."

Veruschka admits that, most of all, she likes looking like a dancer. Setting out to shop for clothes in a city bores her. Often one does not find what one wants, and then it is depressing. Sometimes she has her ideas made up for her, but that takes too much time. So she picks up interesting folklore "shapes" in her wanderings, combines them with city-bought boots and tights and her own long hair and legs.

"The Italians, on the contrary, have a natural elegance," she says. "They don't have much courage, but you never see anyone badly dressed. They instinctively choose a simple chic—good bags, always good shoes, boots, and colors. Italians never disturb you. Only I don't think they have much fun in dressing. Maybe it wouldn't be right for Italian beauties. But at parties, you feel the young people would like to break loose."

Mirella Haggiag agrees with Veruschka about the boredom of much dressing and shopping. She is convinced that not only have the old distinctions about day and evening wear gone out the window (except for gala evenings) but that women really would prefer to have one basic look for all seasons as well. She means a basic covering to wear with sandals in the summer or to throw a fur over when it is cold. This is still a longing more than a reality.

Mirella, too, buys wherever she feels in the mood, then coordinates in Rome. The boots, shoes, and bags are from her home base, as are her pants. Almost all the clothes she really wears are "off the peg" Italian.

"Every time I go to London, I do the boutiques there and come back with scads of what seem to be great finds," she says. "I should know better—I never wear them. My husband has gently pointed out that I can't get away with cheap things. He's right."

And that remark is the crux of the matter. Depending on one's type and year of birth, the costume carnival look spells either enchantment or instant disaster. This holds true whether it is mad boutique and cheap, or ancient and luxurious. Talitha Getty, slender and fragile, with a diaphanous face, would retain her subtlety wrapped in a rag rug. Tall, striking Veruschka would be wasted in conventional gear. I, for one, cannot get away with the folk or far-out approach. It looks too raggy. It may be my inbred Italian sense of moderation protesting, but I feel that most women, particularly those over thirty, do well to eschew it. We have to work a bit harder, organize within a more narrow range, to distill our kind of glamour. Mind you, I no longer think that chic has to be expensive, as I once did. It would never cross my mind now to spend on couture clothes what I did ten years ago. Although when I see a truly superb Valentino collection, I admit, I go straight out of my mind.

Speaking of the total look, Valentino is it to the last perfect detail. His sense of proportion and muted color are infallible. A few tips from the

Italian master designer: "I look first at a woman's shoes," Valentino says. "If they are wrong, her elegance is wrong. Her bag can be carried with a certain nonchalance, but the bag, shoes, and gloves must be perfect. And they must look new." He adds that grooming is all. "The hippie look on women, as opposed to girls, is unforgivable. The love goddess syndrome also kills any real elegance. Overtly sexy women look a mess in clothes."

In my opinion, even a sexy look can be done well. Think of some of the great entertainers and movie stars. But the look, however compelling, has nothing to do with chic or glamour.

In a completely different vein, Britain's Queen Elizabeth has her own distinctive style. You may not find it exciting, but as total looks go, she has one, and anything that integral must be done on purpose.

So where do you go for clothes if your line is neither couture, folklore, royalty, nor love goddess? Like most women these days, I rely on boutiques. My personal choice happens to be classic boutique from Trico, Saint Laurent, or Jean Muir. In the mood for fluff and fun, it is Sant'Angelo, who handles it so deftly. There are so many boutiques, any woman can soon discover which ones suit her best.

Spreading the buying around has its disadvantages, especially in sportswear. You find the pants in one place, the top in another, the scarf in a third, and end up walking miles to get exactly what you want. You cannot eliminate all the trudging about. What you can do is limit its duration. For instance, I set up my wardrobe twice a year. After the boutique collections, I order in late fall for spring and summer and in the spring for fall and winter. Once the clothes are ordered, I concentrate on accessories and separates as soon as they are in the shops, and that more or less does it. (The shops in Rome are Dal Co, Fendi, Gucci.) Between seasons, if I spot something divine when I am downtown for other reasons, I buy it, but I rarely go out just to do shopping.

Consuelo Crespi, who still wears more couture than most women I know, has a similar organizational scheme. "I figure out what I need for the following season right after the high-fashion collections. You have to think ahead and know what you want. After the clothes, I fill in the rest so that every turnout is complete. If you don't organize, not only do you fail to correlate, you wind up spending a lot more on rushed purchases that often are unsatisfactory."

Even Consuelo has cut down on couture, in part because of the tedium of fittings. But she likes her coats and evening clothes to be high fashion, usually Valentino, Mila Schon, or Galitzine.

"Elegance will eventually fade away," she says; "for now it's still irresistible and nice to depend on. I like to mix high fashion with boutique. The all-out 'expensive' look is not right anymore." Consuelo admits that it is far more difficult to dress well now than in the good old days when you went to the favorite couturiers and that was that. The fantasy element has become indispensable. It need not be a total carnival look; it can be a scarf, a choker, a gadget. But without a flair for fantasy, you look dowdy; you have to think of the extras that give clothes a lift.

As for organizing in advance, which seems to me

so indispensable, it can be done even if you cannot attend the collections. The newspapers cover them instantly, followed by the weeklies, and a month or so later, the magazines with photographs and fullest coverage appear. Each publication has an editorial slant, so either you trust one of them, or you buy three or four and make a synthesis. Informed, you can set aside a time just before the major clothes seasons and buy in one coordinated swoop.

A trick of many American businesswomen who have almost no time to shop, yet must look well, is to establish a solid rapport with a buyer in one or two shops they like. The buyer both follows fashion and knows her customer's needs and tastes. She makes a selection. The businesswoman spends a few hours in the shop or has the clothes sent over to her house off-hours for a look-see.

Planning closet space is almost as essential as planning a wardrobe. In order to put clothes together well, you have to be able to see what you have at a glance. Asked for advice on successful living, actress Lillian Gish has been quoted as saying: "Keep your stocking drawer straightened out, and everything will be fine."

Taken symbolically or literally, things have to be kept in order. That old hidden jumble will not do. Ira Furstenberg had rows of perspex drawers designed for her dressing room to give her instant appraisal of her belongings. If not perspex, at least have drawers with window panes. In redoing my dressing room, I replaced drawers with open shelves for easier access. The various items can be placed on them in five-and-dime-store plastic bags.

(That is the weak point in my closetry—I never have enough bags in the right sizes.)

Doing a dressing room is much like doing a bathroom. It would be nice to spend the money elsewhere, but setting them up properly so simplifies one's life, it is well worth the investment. "Accessories have become all-important," Consuelo says, "and so many of them are cumbersome, we have all had to readjust our closets. You have to find room for boots and beads and hats and scarves and shoulder bags—even my evening bags are shoulder bags."

Consuelo and her daughter Pilar wrap magazines around their boots with rubber bands so they will stand straight. Big belts are attached to hangers, as are some of the shoulder bags. Pilar prefers hooks on the walls, and hangs her beads that way, too. No matter how big the bead box or drawer, unless you hang them, beads always tangle. Consuelo's other closet tip: If it's in season and you have not worn it for two months, throw it out. We all have a tendency to keep useless clutter, but more important than the number of things you own is having what one needs well-displayed. When you can see it all at a glance, it gives you ideas for new combinations.

The same technique is valid for packing. I am no authority, but to avoid disastrous oversights, all my clothes are brought out the day I pack. Many of the dresses have their own coats, but I always pack one coat that goes with everything. Shoes and bags go in a separate suitcase. Evening clothes often require matching shoes, but to cut down, I plan my day clothes so that one pair can be worn with various outfits. I also have all-purpose bags, gold for evening, tortoiseshell-colored for day. I know there is a whole mystique about traveling light. On the other hand, if you have to live out of suitcases for six weeks on a business trip just when the season changes, I do not see how you can do it. I am afraid I agree with Valentino. Asked how he packs, he answered, "Oh, I just take lots of clothes."

The paragon of organization is Marella Agnelli. Her beauty, her clothes, her house, her life have inimitable style. "I can be ready to go anywhere in a half hour," she says. "In the beginning, it was difficult, but living with Gianni, it has to be that way." How do you coordinate chic and style with speed and hyperactivity? Marella, both mentally and physically, is an untiring wonder, always ready to explore any new person, idea, or place. More than once, she has told me, "You're so lazy, you make me lazy." As Truman Capote, in a piece for *Vogue*, summed it up: "One first thinks: My God, what a beauty she is! and him. . . . As for her . . . if she should ever invite you to go sight-seeing, or skiing, or shopping, or even for a casual stroll, look her straight in her huge, iridescent, permanently astonished eye and say, 'No, Donna Marella, definitely not!' . . . Let her go. Alone. She will survive. You won't; or scarcely."

First of all, in all her houses, Marella has a *nécessaire* packed, closed, and ready to go. The beauty case, replenished the day of her return, contains all beauty and pharmaceutical products she needs in small, disposable sizes. Secondly, she keeps a basic wardrobe in Rome as well as in Turin and country clothes in their Piedmont place to avoid packing in volume for routine shuttlings.

Thirdly, she, too, plans her fashion in advance, selects the basic colors for the season, and buys in a brief swoop. Her shoes are always low-heeled because she likes to walk as much as possible, even in the city.

Marella's brand of chic last winter was pants and a tunic, a scarf at the neck, and a fur coat for the cold. She almost never wears jewels, though she used to and could get away with enormous hunks that on anyone else would be instant *nouveau riche*. On her, they looked casual.

"Except for evening clothes, I don't buy high fashion anymore," she says. "It's too complicated when you travel as much as I do—for high fashion, you have to take a maid. How simple things have become," she says with relief. "No one is ecstatic anymore about the perfect woman. That era is over."

Marella is a modern rather than a classical beauty, exuding alertness and vitality rather than harmony in repose. Tall and slender, with a proud small head poised on the longest of necks, she keeps her hair simple and short. As for makeup, in her case the less the better. If she made up more, the result might be striking, yet it would also make her conventional. Most of the women she knows are adept at makeup, but few have her quality of feature and bone. Letting her features speak for themselves gives her a look of her own.

"My mother [American Margaret Clarke] was one of the true beauties of her day," Marella says. "She was a cultured woman, but most of her time was spent taking care of herself. She had turquoise eyes and red hair and used to put makeup on even to go to bed. This incessant preoccupation gave me a feeling of anguish. I knew as I grew up that I could never match such beauty. It was useless to concentrate my energy there. Instead, I thought: I'll read, I'll ski, I'll travel."

We do not all have the looks and life of Marella Agnelli, that is for sure. But the idea is to coordinate what we do have and make it work for us. There was a cartoon years ago with two men sprawled in easy chairs, drinks at hand, the picture of disorderly, do-nothing bliss. I may be a word or two off, but in effect, one man says to the other: "We've simply got to get ourselves organized." Well, we all do. There is no chic, no polish, no glamour without organization.

8 *On Being Photogenic*

There are women who always look great in pictures. With or without proper makeup, no matter how amateur the photographer, how awkward the angle, how bad the lighting, they emerge from film victorious. Others come out badly nine times out of ten. Yet such camera disasters are liable to be as good-looking in real life as the photogenic wonders —often they are more beautiful. Why does this happen?

"Some people say they just hate to be photographed. Maybe that's the reason," I once remarked to veteran fashion photographer Joe Leombruno, who has spent twenty-seven successful years in the business with Jack Bodi. "Nonsense," Joe answered. "They love to be photographed. Everyone does, even if they're scared."

Certainly, everyone would like to be photogenic. In this visually conscious world, swamped as we are by images, it is aggravating always to look one's worst on camera. First of all, you cannot escape the lens. Even if you are not in the public eye, friends and relatives are still snapping away. And once in the public eye, you are barraged.

There is one law of compensation. It is no coincidence that the more you are photographed, the better your pictures look. Familiarity with the ever present camera can breed contempt and a frantic desire for privacy, but it also breeds increasing contentment with the photographic results.

Look at the pictures of women suddenly thrown into a limelight they never sought—women made prominent by their own accomplishments or wives of presidents or government leaders. Whether or not they are beauties, they become more photogenic by exposure.

Or take the case of models and actresses for whom beauty is a profession. Again, they get better and better the more their picture is taken. They seem to improve with experience, the way a good wine improves with maturing. (Of course, there is a point of diminishing return—with beauties as with certain wines aged beyond their peak, when the flash or the cork pops, the aroma remains, but the "body" has gone.)

Granted that actresses and models usually start with a face that photographs easily, they learn to perfect this gift. Most of us will never match their professionalism, but what they have to say about the camera is pertinent.

"A model spends more hours in front of a mirror in a year than most women do in a lifetime," former international model Mirella Haggiag explains. "You don't just learn makeup tricks. You learn which muscle lowers the nose or widens the mouth. You learn to use every possibility you have on camera and off. Ultimately, you make of your face whatever you want. In my early pictures, my nose looks wider than it does now. I didn't have surgery—concentration thinned it.

"I rarely do modeling jobs anymore," she continues, "and each time I go back, I'm convinced I won't be as photogenic as before. That's because

I'm out of practice. Being photogenic is like gymnastics—you have to keep at it."

"I can sense instantly if the light is right or wrong when I'm photographed," says Sophia Loren. "I can feel it on my face, and I turn until it's right. If you'd had fourteen years in the business, you would too."

"An actress has to understand her face and body down to the last detail," Virna Lisi declares. "Seeing how you come out on film, you begin to know just where you should be in relation to the camera —three-quarters, to the left, to the right, and so on. In my case, I know that any angle is all right if the hair is fluffy. With the hair pulled back, I have to be more careful. And an actress doesn't learn all by herself. She's surrounded by people whose interest is to advise her."

"If I have to look young, happy, and healthy for a cover," says Veruschka, "and it's a day when I look pale, it takes five minutes. First I put shine on top of the cheekbones to bring them out, a base of light under the eyes on over to the ears, a pink frame around the face, glow and more glow. I look as if I'd been out in the sun and fresh air for weeks.

"The best makeup for photography is theatrical makeup. 'Indio' is fantastic; it comes in any kind of color. There are ten greens. . . ."

But if you are not professional—and most of us are not—the only solution is perhaps the hardest one: Relax, stop worrying about the camera and pretend it isn't there. Be the way you are alone or with good friends. This applies particularly to candid shots, news photographs, and other unexpected exposure. Having a sitting is something else again. There it is the rapport that counts, your confidence in the photographer, and his ability to understand you visually.

Maybe your luck with photography has always been good. You project the image you want without really trying. Perhaps, on the contrary, you look like the wrath. In this case, analyzing bad pictures often reveals where the trouble lies. If it is the lighting or other technical defects, unless being photogenic is your business, blame it on the photographer, but the problem to solve might be you and your face.

The fact is that we are not all born equal in front of the camera. Even women famous for beauty and chic can come out losers. The Duchess of Windsor, for example, has a charm and magnetism that are almost never captured in her pictures. Basically, the photogenic face has wide-set eyes, small features, good cheekbones and jawline, most of which you either inherit or you do not. There are exceptions. Fashion photographer Henry Clarke points out that the late French cover girl Nicole only became a model because she was bound and determined. "While she lived, she was the most popular French model," Henry says. "You couldn't book her. Yet Nicole had no face. She painted it on."

We do not all possess basically photogenic features, nor have the drive of a Nicole, but there is no reason to be camera shy. A good hard look at the pictures you have can be a revelation. It adds up to criticizing yourself as if you were someone else. This is easier with photos than in front of the mirror. Stills bring defects into focus and make them more noticeable than when the face is mobile. Bearing in mind that the camera tends to broaden or flatten the face, what you try to correct for photography usually pays off in real life as well.

Talented young photographer Elisabetta Catalano suggests you look first at the eyebrows. Do they frame the eyes correctly? How about the eye make-up? A few false lashes applied individually can help, whereas too many can seem to close the eye. How are the cheekbones? Do they need shadow underneath and light on the bone to make them exist? Is the makeup excessive? In color shots, this is disaster.

Are you always in the same stance—that dreary one-foot-in-front-of-the-other pose that is supposed to be elegant and usually just looks stiff? What are the hands doing? Are you thrusting your décolleté for all it's worth like a pinup of the forties? (Joe Leombruno says that from the photographer's angle it's wild when all the bosom comes straight at the camera—he does not know whether to grab or dodge.) Do you slump until you look pregnant when sitting? Are your legs crossed so that the top one looks enormous? Is the collar out of propor-tion to your face and height? Does the jewelry look dinky—too much of it and none with a good shape?

If the jawline is dubious, try to avoid being shot from below. Is the profile fantastic? That does not oblige you to be taken in profile for the rest of your life, but it is nice to know it can be counted on. Are smiling shots or serious ones most successful on the average?

Again, you have to think in terms of yourself. The picture evidence is spread out in front of you, and it is on this basis that you work. Imitating the poses models take can be misleading. What is right for their face and body is not necessarily right for any-one else. And being relatively inexperienced, you might imitate the clichés that the best models have abandoned.

But being photogenic is not just features and knowing how to move. You start there because as you discover ways to improve yourself physically, it gives you more assurance and, at bottom, being photogenic is mental.

"I was in Spain recently and photographed two young countesses," Henry Clarke said. "No matter what I did with one of the girls, nothing came out. The other worked like a charm. It must be mental —the first girl was far prettier.

"Once I had dinner and drinks at the house of a marvelous-looking woman in Rome and saw great possibilities," he continued. "It was impossible to photograph her. She looked worried and strained and couldn't relax. Maybe she wanted to be a disaster. She told me her photos never were any good."

Relaxing in front of the camera, if you do not spend much of your life there, can be difficult. It is for me. But as Henry suggests, if you cannot relax, for heaven's sake, take a tranquilizer before the shooting starts. Put on a record, have a drink. Most good photographers do their best to put you at ease. After all, they want good pictures, too. There can be incompatibility between photographer and subject—in any field, you get along better with some people than others. But when a sitting has been arranged, it is in a professional's interest to do the best possible job.

"Good photographs are 50 percent subject and 50 percent photographer," says Joe Leombruno.

"But it's 100 percent the photographer's fault if nothing comes across. He has to know how to handle people and do it gently. Sometimes the subjects who freeze are the nicest ones. If you're getting nowhere, you take a break, have a coffee, talk for a while."

I do not know Cecil Beaton personally and have never been photographed by him. From what I understand, when he does portraits, he moves about so quietly, his presence is inaudible. The subject is never pressured—there seems to be all the time and leisure in the world. Meanwhile, one can be sure that nothing, but nothing, escapes the Beaton eyes.

As I mentioned previously, Dick Avedon photographed me on two separate occasions and the pictures were never accepted by the magazines. Maybe I am not his type. He does seem to excel at making rather unusual women look fabulous. Perhaps it's mood or time—both sessions were at the end of long, arduous days. Dick, whom many call the greatest photographer of our age, has pioneered many new techniques and prefers studio work to straight reportage—he has that unique ability to climb inside a woman's personality and project it back through the camera.

I recall Dick saying at the beginning of our second session, "I must tell you quite honestly you were very dull ten years ago—now I have got you"; but the pictures still didn't strike the editor's fancy. Oh well, now that I am a member of the family, perhaps I will get a third chance.

In addition to having a relaxed, natural attitude —helped in this by the photographer—being photogenic is mental in another way. If you are an interesting person and interested in many things, this shows in the eyes and the expression of the mouth. And it shows instantly in the camera to a sensitive lens man.

Buxy Gancia, who has worked on both sides, as a model who started with Chanel and as an occasional photographer for fashion magazines, says that any woman who can produce an expression can be photogenic.

"It's the inside salt that counts," she claims. "If you have it, the photographer should sense it, and don't let him push you around. If you're not a fashion model, there's no sense trying to look like one. And anyhow, today we're in a period where faults become charm. You can have freckles and an impossible little nose and still be divine in pictures."

There is even a trend today to have models look like "people" rather than anonymous perfections or vehicles for all those gorgeous clothes. Many a fashion photographer can tell you there is a glut of highly trained models who are impossible to use anymore because they are specialized morons.

The same trend prevails in films, where the plus-perfect superstar and love goddess no longer stirs anyone under seventy. Look at the female leads in the more exciting films by young directors. They may not look like the girl next door—why should they when they lead a different life?—but in the main they are irregular, imperfect beauties. This does not stop them from being photogenic; in fact, it makes their image more involving and far more moving—you sense a few quirks under the skin.

A forerunner in this direction, as in countless other movie trends, is director Michelangelo

Antonioni. When he casts a film, his only concern is that the actors and actresses look right to him for the roles they have to play. Nothing else matters. It is up to the cameraman to light them properly and make them photogenic.

No one believed, for example, that Monica Vitti would photograph well enough for movies. That is, no one did until she played the lead in Antonioni films.

"I don't know one rule, criterion, or norm for being photogenic," the director says. "It's a mystery to me. And I have no patience at all with stars who tell me what side they should be photographed from. I couldn't care less about their better profile."

Yet the women in Antonioni films have great intensity. In part, this may be because he gives them credible roles to play, both understanding the complexity of any real woman and preferring it to stereotypes. His women are always beautiful, which is what we are primarily concerned with here— each one in a particular, personal way. Granted he is visually aware to a degree that even few directors attain, I assume his women all had something to begin with or he would not have seen it. The rest is direction and bringing the beauty out. An actress trusts Antonioni—and who would not? For his part, Antonioni gives an actress her head. His instructions are rarely detailed.

No matter how formal or casual the occasion, photography always takes this sort of collaboration. The director or the man with the camera has to react to you and you to him. Preferably, you get along. If you can respect each other, talk and laugh together, the results are apt to be better.

"Don't look on a sitting as a bad situation," advises Ugo Mulas, Italy's leading all-around photographer. "Try not to give a damn. If you know he's a good photographer, trust him and let him work. If you don't like him, throw him out."

Often you cannot choose the photographer, much less throw him out, if the pictures are for the press. (You can, but it makes an unpleasant scene.) Often the photographer is assigned and cannot choose his subjects. If he had his choice, there are a lot of people he would rather not do, that is for sure. So in a way, both of you are trying to bail out the same boat.

When the pictures are for a leading magazine, or for an advertisement, there is a pre-photography session to get everyone organized. The editor and photographer will go through your wardrobe to choose the best turnouts for the spread. Whether or not you want a hairdresser or makeup man for the occasion is cleared in advance. (The main exception here is royalty. In that case, the photographer and editor have to take what they can get. Farah Diba has been known to let a photographer choose what he thinks she would photograph best in. Most members of royalty do not—although it might be to their advantage.)

Working with a personality, as opposed to a pro, is always more of a challenge to a photographer. The personality is not bred to the camera—the skills lie in other areas. You may be nervous, but so is the magazine or newspaper team until the setting goes smoothly. You want to know whether you look well or not. They want to know whether or not they have a spread that can be published. Yet, despite basically good mutual intentions, in self-defense you have to learn something about the business if you are in a position to be photographed frequently. This is especially true when you are being photographed for your looks.

"I've often been badly done," says fashion magazine and women's editor favorite Talitha Getty. "They ask you to assume certain positions, tell you 'yes, yes, hold it,' and you come out ridiculous. I'm no professional, but I'm beginning to know what's good and what's bad. My nose is fairly long, and I've learned, for instance, that if my face is down when I laugh, all you see in the picture is nose and a huge smile. It still makes me nervous to work with a photographer I don't know and trust."

"I despise being photographed," says Marella Agnelli. "That will never change." (And to the end, she will go on looking elegant and distinguished in her pictures, with a hint of the humor that photographers find so refreshing in her.)

I must say that I, for one, am no example to hold up to others facing the camera. It is not all that easy to photograph me. I have learned through experience that certain hairstyles do not work and that my profile is best. But every time I have to have pictures taken, I am convinced I have not learned a thing. In the beginning, it is a great thrill to see that you can look beautiful. But you are never really sure. To my mind, it all depends on the photographer.

The ones I do not know always make me nervous. Sometimes we click—in five minutes—you can sense when a sitting is going well. Often, it takes much longer.

It helps to try and get an idea of either the photographer's style or that of the magazine before posing. This is to protect yourself. With a good photographer, you take his lead, collaborate, and try to have a pleasant time of it. (If he happens to be good and your boyfriend to boot, then you are really protected, but in most cases with models, to say nothing of personalities or the photographers themselves, such rapport is extraneous to the matter at hand.)

Confronted with a poor professional or one of the distortion fiends, you have to be careful or they destroy you. If a photographer puts you in a position that is uncomfortable, refuse it because it will look awkward. Watch out for close-ups in which every pore comes out a crater and every line a ditch. All photographers should be taught not to make people look horrible, but there are phases and fads in the business when this is fashionable. Just make sure it is not at your expense. You do not care about having a trendy picture. You want to look well.

"I don't like cruel photography," Henry Clarke says. "The wide-angle lens for portraits is dishonest, focusing on a wart is dishonest. I think all those boys are out to prove something, but they are not taking pictures of human beings.

"This doesn't mean you take everyone through a soft lens, embowered in tulle and roses. The aim is to capture their look and personality. When Chanel made her comeback, I took a straight picture of her. She came out a marvelous, tough old girl with a lot of chic, which is what she is. She didn't look like a monster—she isn't one—the man behind the camera is, if he purposely takes her at bad angles."

To put it in another way, listen to one of photography's greats, Henri Cartier-Bresson. He does not do fashion and glamour—that is not his world. The exterior-interior rapport, the expression that for an instant conveys the underlying and surrounding reality, is what he wants to capture. His faces have the beauty of truth. And no one more abhors artifice, distortion, contrived angles, and gimmicks.

When he can, Cartier-Bresson works without identifying himself, as if he were just another tourist snapping away with a Leica. When he does portraits, he cannot be anonymous, but his technique, as in reportage, is ". . . velvet paws and a sharp eye. No agitation; you don't stir up the water before you fish." He prefers to do people in their own ambiance, even though he knows that the simple presence of a photographer and his equipment already conditions what he calls the "victim."

As he wrote in the preface to *Photographies de H-C-B*: "There is a certain parentage in all the portraits done by the same photographer because his understanding of people is linked to his own psychological structure. Harmony is refound by looking for the equilibrium in the asymmetry of every face. This avoids suavity or the grotesque."

If the best of the truth photographers finds that putting people at a disadvantage with the camera is dishonest, I do believe there is no sense going along with lesser craftsman's fun and games. If you are not extremely photogenic, find out who it is who wants to take pictures, particularly for publication, and act accordingly.

On the other hand, I confess that, much as I dislike the grotesque, I am rather in favor of suavity in pictures of me. I am not purist—nasty lies, no; little white ones, yes. I want to be flattered. Most women do because most of us neither are

Greta Garbo nor convey overwhelming soul. I think I have made it clear that much of our look on film is up to us. The rest, if we candidly state that our aim is to be as attractive as possible, becomes the photographer's job, be he amateur or professional.

9 Beauty and the Astrologers

Most of us believe in astrology a little, and some of us quite a lot. I, for one, am not so foolish as not to believe. If I have weighed the pros and cons and am really convinced about something, I will go ahead and do it—but weighing the pros and cons might well include a trip to the fortune-teller as well as to the astrologer.

I never know whether the advice of the astrologer is inevitable or whether one is so influenced by the advice that this actually makes the prediction come true. Talitha Getty once confessed she never had her horoscope done: "I made hundreds of appointments and never showed up. I was always too afraid." Years ago an old Roman friend, Prince Dado Ruspoli, told me that my marriage would be over in six months. I was very surprised at the time, but Dado, much interested in astrology, was certain. Six months later, my husband and I separated.

Anyone who has studied astrology can make surface observations on the beauty attributes of any sign. I am a Capricorn and so a slow starter whose beauty improves with age. Scorpios are sensuous with magnetic eyes. Sagittarians have good legs and are at their best with a casual chic. Aries are dynamos—no one does the sports look better. Leos are proud beauties who need adulation to thrive, while Aquarians thrive simply by being out of doors. Virgos are almost too well groomed, with never a hair out of place, and Geminis have good bodies but much prefer dialogue to beauty care. Libras are the natural beauties and Cancer girls tend to put on weight. Pisces take well to the water but their fair skin cannot take the sun. Taurus's sign always means an early splendor and a great fight later against excess weight.

Does all this mean that your beauty type is always inherent in your astrological sign? It depends on one's personal attitude toward astrology. Pure zodiac types are rare—not every Taurus man has a bull neck; not every Libra is a ravishing beauty. Your ascendant (the sign rising at the time of birth) will usually modify your natal sign, and the total configuration of the chart comes into play. Whether you can or cannot describe a person accurately merely by knowing their sign is not really important here; what is important is that astrology can often serve admirably to illuminate your character. And once past your twenties, character plays a larger part in keeping your beauty than anything you were born with.

A Capricorn's life, for example, is a long determined trudge up a mountain. The peak may always be in view but Capricorns sometimes feel they will never reach it. They are perfectionists and hence often depressed by their failure to reach perfection. I used to fight these sieges of depression. I would refuse to admit that there was anything wrong and I would wind up looking a wreck. Now that I know, through astrology, that it isn't only me, that all Capricorns are prone to down periods, instead of fighting, I try to ride them out, resting and lying low as much as possible. The result is that the blues seem to end more quickly and now occur far less often.

If you follow newspaper horoscopes (and who can resist them, despite knowing they cannot possibly apply to everyone), it seems that all sorts of adventurous, romantic things are predicted every day, except when you get to Capricorn. There it is always work, work, work. Maybe that is why I am convinced that being active is good for beauty. As a Capricorn, I am doomed to it.

There is one consolation, at least as far as I am concerned: The work is rarely housework. I have never been any good at it, and now I can say it is fate. If you want "the angel in the house," the woman whose place is in the home, do not marry a Capricorn. The hearth is not their scene. They can organize and entertain well. Put them to sewing buttons and washing dishes and they look like eighty after a month and the buttons tend to fall right off again.

Apart from helping you to understand your own character and how to take care of yourself, a knowledge of astrology can make you more tolerant of others. This, too, as you know, cuts down on stress, which causes wear and tear on the nerves. Somehow it is easier to live with other people's defects when you can attribute them to a sign. A man's messiness, flight from responsibility, and lack of financial sense may be just as chronic as they ever were, but knowing he is a Pisces gives the traits a sort of cosmic inevitability. It is probably too late to change him. So instead of breaking out into a rash and developing a forehead resembling a furrowed field, you try to look to your own stars and overlook his. (Mind you, he is bound to have some of those good Pisces qualities as well.)

For example, Emilio Pucci is a Scorpio. "Isn't it obvious?" he asks. "Women born under the sign have even more sexuality than the men, although they may be less aware of it. Happily, they also possess mental qualities—it's a formidable combination. If, like my wife, you're Gemini, at times you just cannot do things. She is capable of turning around and going home again on her way to the airport. To illustrate the difference between us: I suffer from sinus, and if I've been at a party where lots of people smoke, I wake up the next morning with excruciating pain—nonetheless, I get up. On the other hand, my wife can be so upset if breakfast is late, she has to go back to bed. I realize now it's not caprice—she's a Gemini."

Rudi Crespi, a Leo, adores the sun and lies motionless on the sand six hours at a time. Leos are also known to take good care of themselves, and Rudi not only uses a good cream when he comes in from the sun, he tries to have a skin checkup by Dr. Norman Orentreich once a year to ward off ill effects. Does Rudi believe in astrology? Every month he reads astrologers Waldner, Celeste, and Prové, compares them, and does his own chart. Then he does his family's in relation to himself. Consuelo, his wife, is another Gemini, but the split personality, considered to be typical of the sign, has another dimension here. After years as wife, mother, and hostess, she shifted gears and became a professional journalist. And there must be other stars at work or a stabilizing ascendant—as a journalist, you meet deadlines, catch planes, and keep appointments.

Most of the beautiful Italians I know believe in some form of cosmic harmony or the occult—astrology, cycles, handwriting, clairvoyance, ESP, yoga, or hara. This does not mean they are necessarily against science or, should they need it, psychiatry. The fact is they enjoy the marginal disciplines and seem to look the better for it. A common practice among them is to burn incense, sandalwood, or perfume in the house. Whether or not the hostess modestly protests it is just to clear the air, everyone knows it is also done to create good vibrations. The perfume always emanates from a carefully chosen place in the room and a certain ritual surrounds the performance. The choice of the scent itself is a form of aromato-therapy. Certain odors relax or stimulate us, making us feel more beautiful.

And even those who scoff at the occult use herbs in food, unconsciously assimilating a long tradition of magic. They may not know why they use them, except for flavor, but their grandmothers knew. The basil they tuck into sauces and salads favors love. Chewing anise wards off the evil eye, and bay leaves, favored by the Delphic priestesses, protect against witches and Satan. Keyholes and cracks were once stuffed with fennel against evil spirits. For all I know, eating raw fennel as Italians do, dipped in olive oil, salt, and pepper, may have the same effect.

As for herbs with aphrodisiac properties, surely they embody beauty magic. Mint, for example, is fed to bulls and stallions to strengthen them, and rosemary used to be given to the bridegroom before the wedding night. Soup flavored with thyme also spurs lust. To reinforce honey's aphrodisiac value, Sheikh Nefzawi in *The Perfumed Garden* suggests a broth of purified honey and onion juices. The Roman poet Martial also firmly believed in the onion: "If your wife is old and your member is exhausted, eat onions in plenty." And garlic (if both of you eat it) is said to be even more conducive than onion. Nicholas Culpepper, the famous herbalist, defines its heat as "vehement." Culpepper attributes the power of various herbs to the planets, which brings us back to astrological signs.

Industrialist Nino Cerruti, dark-haired and startlingly good-looking, is in textiles and boutiques. Granted the textile business was in the family, but fashion is an ideal occupation for beauty-loving Libras, and one simply could not imagine him in coal mining or manufacturing garbage cans. "I'm Libra with a Libra ascendant," he says. "I believe in it up to a point. Of course, I love what is beautiful, but culture or an intelligent attitude are indispensable, especially for the rich. If a woman feels less ugly having a face-lift, that is fine. Personally, I'd rather see the money spent on giving people who need it a chance to grow up well."

Any astrologer would quickly note that this is the Libra sense of justice coming out. Cerruti's therapy for fatigue—long, soothing, tepid baths—is another Libra trait.

"I'm a perfect Aquarius," says fashion world's Mirella Haggiag. "I'm very anxious and I live for the future. The past doesn't exist and the present, just barely. I write long memos to myself about things to do."

"I'm Aquarius, born at midday, and I feel very Aquarius," says Franco Zeffirelli. "But you know, I'm Florentine and very proud of my Tuscan balance. Anything that might make me lose it is suspicious. I shy away from cults and the convoluted, abstract levels that modern culture is heading toward. When I grew up, Copenhagen didn't exist because my father hadn't been there. What wasn't experienced directly had no reality."

On the other hand, perhaps because of his balance, Franco believes in cycles. (So do astrologers.) He says he was lucky for many years and it all came naturally. Two years ago, he sensed he should stop and take a holiday in the Far East. Not for any mystic reasons, he protests, only because he had never been there. He did not take the vacation. First he was in a bad accident (with Gina Lollobrigida, driving to Florence for a soccer game), then two scripts aborted and other projects failed to develop. He is only beginning to come out from under now.

I confess the cycle theory can be compelling. Cristina Ford was eight years married, eight years alone. I was eight years married, eight years alone. And may we both live happily ever after!

Prince Dado Ruspoli, who predicted the breakup of my marriage, was attracted to the occult when he was seventeen. He began with spiritism, which he gave up because of the fear of forces one cannot control. He still retains a certain clairvoyance—he celebrated the day of his son's conception, absolutely sure it was that day and not another, by a baptismal ceremony with the four elements. "We were in St. Tropez, so we started with water," he said. "I predicted my son would be born on May 31. Three days before that date, the gynecologist said it was impossible. On May 31, my wife, using the discipline of hara, had the baby by natural childbirth."

His wife, Nancy, still does astrology, but he does less of it now. While still very much engrossed, he told Sophia Loren, after she lost her second child in Rome, that she would have a child within a year, but with a different doctor. Sophia had her son and did indeed change doctors.

Dado, who has traveled extensively in the Orient, now is much taken with zen and Japanese hara. (Aries, his sign, favors impulsive, changing enthusiasms and great curiosity.) He wears a medal engraved with a buddha that was given him by a monk in the north of Thailand. The monk told him that he would have an accident on a certain day. Dado had a tattoo done so that the accident would be bloodless and did not go out the day the accident was to occur. At 9 P.M., however, an Italian Embassy car came to take him to a dinner he had forgotten. Dado refused the car, but as he could not refuse the invitation, took a rickshaw instead. A taxi knocked the rickshaw over, fracturing two of his ribs. He asked the monk how he could have known about the accident. The monk stated that life is like a river, and you cannot see beyond the bend. However, said the monk, "I'm up in a tree."

The book that has had the greatest influence on Dado recently is Graf Karlfried von Durckheim's *Hara, Man's Vital Center*. Hara, in simplified terms, has to do with finding one's center of balance, the lower abdomen, and developing it through proper exercise, breathing, and posture. Push a Westerner from behind and, concentrated as he is on the upper regions of the body, he may topple. Push a Japanese, and his conscious center of gravity in the abdomen, his sense of hara, keeps him on keel.

Dado is convinced that plumpness in the hara manner is a form of beauty. Pregnant women have it to the limit, as do most Gothic statues of women, but Dado points out that, strangely enough, the contemporary mannequin's walk is based on it (shoulders down and pelvis thrust forward). "Aside from Buddhas," he says, "look at the men in our world who have had a sphere of influence —Napoleon, Churchill, De Gaulle—and you find hara."

Obviously, for anyone so absorbed in special disciplines, one's beauty is only as durable as one's sense of self and place in the world. I am not as smitten as Dado by oriental wisdoms. You probably are not either. Rather than hara, give me a good gym instructor. I think that, along with self-knowledge, you need all the beauty knowledge you can get to look your best, but the two are linked. If an acquaintance with astrology reinforces your character, your looks can benefit.

One of the obvious correlates of undeveloped character is a face that sags prematurely. I was at a party once where an actress in her forties agreed to be hypnotized. As she went into hypnosis, her face fell. It was her character, her drive to succeed, that had kept her face up all those years. I saw her recently and, in its way, her face is still up.

Some signs seem to denote an innate physical intelligence. For example, Dado points out, when Brigitte Bardot (a Libra) began her career, no one took her seriously. At most, she had the appeal of a Pekinese. She was competing at the time with another standard of beauty—women like Ava Gardner and Liz Taylor. But the little Pekinese, rather than try to be what she was not, imposed her looks as one might impose an idea that was right for the time.

A knowledge of astrology helps in other ways. It

makes us pay attention to the little things, the small acts that make up a day and reveal special quirks and charms: a Libra spending what seems to be endless hours in the bath, a Virgo straightening a crooked painting on the wall, a Taurus' inflexible habits. (Valentino, a Taurus, cannot sleep if his bedroom slippers are not in the precise position he prefers by his bed. He confesses he is very punctilious in his living habits. Sublimated in his couture, this mania for exact detail gives his collections their polished perfection. For that matter, his own looks are impeccable.)

As Dado stresses—and I agree—big events happen only once a year or maybe four times in a life, and they seem to fall on top of us. On the other hand, we can control the little things. In personal beauty terms, we can cultivate a style, do what has to be done every day to preserve and refine it. We cannot look like a Libra if we are Aries, but we can be an Aries that is stupendous.

An awareness of the little things keeps us alert, tones the muscles and puts light in the eyes. If you ask most adults to get a book from a shelf, the process is automatic. If you ask a child, it may take considerably longer. There is so much to see and touch and discover on the way. That, too, is youthfulness.

Astrology will not teach you much about yourself you do not already know. But it might make you more aware of what you know. It could indicate, for example, that your daughter is prone to love at first sight or is attracted by men who are her inferiors. You could help guard her against the stress and heartbreak this often involves.

Astrology, too, could indicate that you tend to

base your life on a man and, without his devotion, grow haggard and unwell. Putting all your emotional eggs in one basket is a risky business, and you would be wise at least to calculate the risk.

Your chart might also confirm your vocation or indicate new possibilities. As a Capricorn, with a Gemini ascendant, work with the public that entails travel turns out to be good for me—in more ways than one. (Though when I've lived out of suitcases for six weeks, I sometimes wonder.) According to the chart a young American, Patricia Norelli-Bachelet, drew up for me a few years ago, the important men in my life are from different countries and often met through travel. My best type of work, due to certain aspects and parallels, is one that deals with finery, luxury, and beautiful objects. When I started to work, I instinctively turned toward beauty and fashion because they are what I know best. Still, it was reassuring to see them in the horoscope.

On the other hand, it is not as if I have achieved perfect harmony. There are still plenty of faults to overcome: restlessness, inconstancy, and a tendency to have too many superficial interests. Miss Bachelet wrote that I have to cultivate my will to the maximum. Certainly, this is true with regard to looks. Without willpower, I could be in bad shape fast. You may have more natural discipline—I have to make a point of it.

Many people consult their astrologer before making any decisions about financial deals, contracts, trips, schools for their children, new jobs, change of residence, pregnancy, cosmetic surgery, anything important. If it puts their mind at rest (and guarantees their beauty sleep), more power to them. Personally, I prefer to avoid this sort of dependency. Specific predictions can play strange tricks on you. Once a famous Roman astrologer told me I was apt to lose something very precious the following month. I rushed out and heavily insured my jewels, furs, and other valuables. It cost a fortune. By the middle of the next month, I was on edge and sleeping badly. My face and nerves were a wreck. So the stars proved true; I lost my favorite man of the moment.

My advice is to enjoy astrology, not become a slave to it—enjoy its form and poetry and symbolism. Marvel at what it can reveal and look on it as one more road to self-perfection. The very fact of being attracted to any sphere of the occult means that it corresponds to a personal need. So by all means indulge. If astrology helps you to be yourself, to do what you like and be with the people you find most compatible, this is a great beauty boost.

As for more specific observations on the beauty-astrology relationship, bear in mind that most of us are mixed types, born under one sign with an ascendant in another. The ascendant, the sign rising on the Eastern horizon at the time of birth, strongly influences our physical appearance, the way people see us. For an astrologer to determine the ascendant, you must know not just the day, but the time you were born. The natal sign, nonetheless, is the basic foundation.

The observations, listed below, were made by astrologers Lucia Alberti, friend and mentor of myriad Romans in the art, literature, show business, and social world, and Francesco Waldner of international fame, whose columns have given him a rather staggering following. It has been estimated that half the adult population in France consults his column in *Elle* magazine.

ASTROLOGY AND BEAUTY

In the astrological tradition, there is less force in the roots of the hair when the moon wanes, because the moon influences all growth. In consequence, hair should be cut when the moon is in the ascendant phase. When falling hair is a problem, the best time for a cut is during the last three days of the full moon. The same rules apply to manicures and pedicures, although nails, which are not expected to grow so much, are less affected.

As for losing weight, Waldner suggests that the best times are when the moon is in Taurus or the sun is in an earth sign. Specifically, it is easiest to resist hunger and eliminate drink in April and May or August and September. These, again, are the best months to change diet or try regimens such as vegetarianism. Any change often improves looks because the liver must work differently.

ZODIACAL TYPES

By Lucia Alberti   *By Francesco Waldner*

ARIES

Very impulsive and emotional; always falling madly in love; alert, curious, and avant-

Very dynamic and active, highly developed senses;
needs rest to avoid ner-

garde; needs rest because of strong emotions; is strong but tends to abuse health, is prone to headaches;
must avoid eyestrain and should not do night work; must have frequent dental checkups.

vous strain and gauntness, facials to relax face; is impatient about beauty care and cannot stand spending hours at the hairdresser; features, however, are often strong and lessons in makeup to balance them are helpful; moderation with alcohol and cigarettes is indicated; eyestrain should be avoided; flair for fashion usually lies either in sportive or "ethnic" looks, such as caftans, Far West.

TAURUS

Beautiful eyes and good skin; very patient, very tenacious, but feels inferior and worries about saying or doing the wrong thing; very possessive in love because needs security; also loves to possess beautiful things— clothes, jewels, furnishings—and should marry man of means; often has a beautiful voice; tends to overeat and must watch diet.

A great beauty when young; tends to put on weight and age quickly, figure must be watched early to avoid this; a creature of habit and must make an effort not to get in rut: should change makeup, hair, and way of dressing from time to time to counteract tendency to overweight; saunas and swimming also are effective; loves the sun and tans well.

GEMINI

Nervous type of beauty with dry skin that must be nourished;
tends to become neurotic and age badly because of dispersed energy and the strain of doing ten things at once, without finishing any of them;
restlessness often leads to discontent and the strained look of discontent;
nerves often make them smoke too much.

Usually intellectual, preferring ideas to beauty treatments;
should perfect a casual style that is suitable to type;
often the face is too long and the nose too long or big—Geminis often resort to cosmetic surgery and many of them must be dissuaded from wanting not just correction, but a nose too tiny for their face;
rarely victims of passion; a man must appeal to their minds, as well as their hearts;
almost always, the body is good and looks last well into maturity.

CANCER

Beautiful eyes;
hypersensitive and insecure, afraid of the future and nostalgic about childhood;
marries young and is attracted to unusual, often unscrupulous men;
much charm when complimented and secure;
is gourmet, but must watch tendency to put on weight when older;

Beautiful when young, develops early, often has interesting eyes;
feminine softness and gentleness very appealing to men;
although should not be too thin, loves to eat and drink and, unless restraint is exercised, starts to put on weight as grows older;
tends to be lazy about

is prone to psychoso-
matic disorders but
retains adolescent ap-
peal until late in life.

beauty and should be
encouraged to make the
effort;
is habit-loving rather
than avant-garde, loath
to discard out-of-date
clothes, makeup and
hairstyles;
suffers from insomnia;
needs saunas, swim-
ming, and sun to keep
body in shape.

LEO

Proud, vain, volatile,
ambitious, extremely
extroverted, and full of
vitality;
noticeably fashionable
with a love for jewelry;
usually has lots of long
hair, very attractive to
men;
tends to marry for pres-
tige, but often has
highly successful career
and is not interested in
marriage;
if ambitions not fulfilled,
can have difficult meno-
pause, wearing clothes
that are too youthful
and low-cut, dyeing her
hair brassy blond or red.

Beautiful when young;
very proud of looks and
takes great care, but can
be obsessed if her hair
is not right or she has
gained two pounds;
preoccupation with looks
can lead to nervous
fatigue;
pay her compliments and
she sleeps well that
night; slight or insult
her, she cannot sleep;
is faithful and cannot
tolerate unfaithfulness;
loves the sun and sports,
usually has beautiful
body.

VIRGO

Remains surprisingly
youthful despite hypo-

Highly organized and
always knows just what

chondriac tendency;
when beautiful is a per-
fectionist about beauty;
but when lonely,
although always clean
and orderly, can neglect
her looks;
tends, like Greta Garbo,
to wear little makeup
and dress with sobriety;
is cerebral, hard worker;
needs affection, but
never falls head over
heels in love.

to wear;
it would be good for her
to be more casual and
relaxed;
perfectionism often is a
cause of insomnia;
has good skin and often
a very cool, collected
beauty that ages
superbly.

LIBRA

The natural beauty with
natural elegance and
equilibrium;
beautiful eyes and a
well-proportioned body;
takes good care of
herself;
rarely gets fat;
very sociable, somewhat
snobbish, loves to flirt
and to please;
detests solitude and a
good marriage is indis-
pensable—while sharp
on the defensive, she is
not enough of a fighter
to go it on her own;
often tires or becomes ill,
but has surprising
recuperative power;
alcohol and cold are her
enemies.

The true young beauty;
adores and is very good
at beauty and fashion,
always avoiding jarring
extremes and fads, has
innate style;
gets up tired and really
wakes up in the after-
noon, needs much rest—
after thirty-six, should
watch weight;
spa cures benefit her
skin, makeup is bad for
it, and proper cleansing
a must;
loves to spend hours in
the bathroom (but may
forget about the ring
around the tub—
although personally
well-groomed, is a bit
untidy about the house);

is extremely diplomatic
and knows how to
handle men;
often more intelligent
than she appears.

SAGITTARIUS

Tall and beautiful;
enthusiasm keeps her
young, independent,
and truthful;
is torn between attrac-
tion to bright, amusing
men who are good
talkers and her desire for
a solid social position;
needs active life and lots
of fresh air;
must watch weight after
forty.

Prefers ideas and talk to
beauty and chic;
tends to put on weight
as matures, but has good
body and usually is
good at sports;
loves traveling, animals,
flowers, and is best with
a casual style;
house a bit cluttered,
but with interesting,
appealing things.

SCORPIO

Interesting type, can be
very seductive;
the face has a diabolical
charm, often looks old
when young and young
when old;
tends to smoke and
drink in excess;
hypersexual and often
attracted to men who are
her inferiors—Scorpios
are the girls who run off
with the chauffeurs;
intensely intelligent,

Extraordinary eyes and
intensity of gaze, great
personal magnetism;
remains young, but can
have cycles in which
looks alternately vibrant
and worn out;
needs rest, but is an
afternoon-night person;
must have varied, active
life;
regular sex life is indispensable to beauty (the
men of the sign remain

takes everything seriously; suffers from anguish.

virile until ripe old age —the classic story is that of the exasperated woman who had two lovers; the young one who attracted her was cold, whereas the seventy-six-year-old Scorpio was always ready); loves drama and, when in form, prefers bright colors; when depressed, wears dark ones; needs yoga or gym because of high-pitched life and spas to eliminate toxins and clear the skin.

Capricorn

Always looks younger than age; either is indifferent to beauty and fashion or is perfectionist; style is understated with little makeup; hates to waste time in idle chatter, but likes to entertain interesting people; absolute need of privacy and a few hours to herself every day; rarely puts on weight; hates publicity, noise,

Slow starter who improves with age; always well turned-out and insists on quality in clothes; extremely well organized; needs yoga or gym for equilibrium; often hides beauty or does not know how to show it to best advantage (counseling could help here); needs to work for well-being.

exhibitionism;
cerebral and needs to
work; must guard
against depression.

AQUARIUS

Interesting-looking, slender; often slightly neurotic and with fragile health; always avant-garde in interests, fashion, and looks; constantly preoccupied with the future; diversified interests and has a career; independent in love, usually finds the right man late; yoga excellent for her nerves.

Another slow starter who improves with age; lots of fresh air and walking indicated as tonic for nerves; because of nervous energy, rarely gets fat; highly personal, inventive taste in fashion, often creates new trends; adores ornament, chains, beads, loves to travel, and often prefers foreign men.

PISCES

One of the zodiac beauties—must watch weight as matures and requires fresh air and sport to reinforce health; tends to overindulge in tranquilizers, pep pills, alcohol, and cigarettes; feet are weak point and pedicures essential; emotionally unstable, must avoid mistaking compassion and pity for

Tends to be lazy and neglectful about beauty and must overcome this; also, must watch weight when mature—swimming and saunas are beneficial; fantasy and imagination give great charm; men also attracted because of sensuousness; pretends to be defenseless, underneath is

love;
has beautiful skin but
must protect it from the
sun.

tenacious.

10 Men

Once again, men's looks are coming into their own. For generations we were brainwashed with the idea that they were not supposed to matter. A woman was expected to be attractive, but as long as a man was intelligent or rich, he could be a monster. We would love him for his talent, his soul, or his bank account. It never worked, of course. Or maybe it did as long as women were not supposed to like making love—as long as they endured it as one more household chore. ("I lie on my back and think of England," the lady explained.)

I am not knocking talent or soul, even if they are not always easy to live with, and certainly I have never had anything against a man being rich. That is good for any woman. What a shame it is that beautiful men rarely have major-league money, because I do like beautiful men—their looks do matter, just as a man's being a good lover is important. (The two are linked unless you live in the dark.)

I once spent a weekend in the country with a man who I was sure was the love of my life. When I saw the mess the place was in, for three days, much as I loathe housework, I wiped, dusted, and scrubbed floors. I am always on edge in country houses, terrified there are not enough locks. As I went about my work, I had visions of being strangled with the vacuum cleaner while my boy friend was strolling the grounds. After the long weekend was over, he decided I was the woman of his life. I decided what he really wanted was a servant. Deliver me from a slob in the house. But at least he was attractive.

Most men now are very conscious about keeping in shape. It is drummed into them for health as well as esthetic reasons. The new clothes require it. Toiletry products and cosmetic surgery further the effort. And women benefit by it. We have the same pleasure in seeing a gorgeous man that men have with a pretty woman.

All the jokes about unisex and not being able to tell the difference are nonsense. I can tell when I want to—and I bet you do not have any trouble either. If with some of the great-looking couples, you are hard-pressed to decide which of the two has the more allure, that is the way it should be.

I might mention in passing that Italian men are not my favorites, but that is a long story and has nothing to do with their looks. (A lot of Italian men, for their part, prefer foreign women. It seems to balance off.) I find most of them are like the bird that is always killed when it sings—so full of itself, it does not hear the hunter coming.

Italian men, if not convinced themselves in their heart of hearts, have perpetrated the myth that they are irresistible—encouraged in this, right from the start, by their mamas. No doubt about it, they are handsome and proud of it. When the new emphasis on men's looks began, they were right in the vanguard.

"If they often get dropped, as Henry James would say, 'it's the blankness,'" comments Gore Vidal. "But they like themselves. They never had that northern puritan thing about the woman being the beauty and the man dirty and ugly."

The handsome Italians in this chapter are among my favorites. They would be on any list. They happen to be very bright, very talented, most of them monied—and all of them devastatingly attractive. (The age range is mid-thirties to mid-fifties, when many of their peers have already gone to beef or fallen apart.) They are far too busy to concentrate on their looks, but they do take care of themselves. And how!

Gianni Agnelli, commenting once on a mother and daughter (in the former's favor), said it was like the difference between champagne and beer. The comparison holds for Gianni and other men. He happens to have everything, including Fiat. He is not good-looking in the classic sense—he has glitter. He can throw on an old towel on a boat or an old sweater at home and still be divine. The looks have character, too, but that would be expected.

Cold showers, engines revved, phones ringing, Gianni has a nonstop attitude toward life that would devastate me, to say nothing of most men I know. Waiting is out of the question. If he had to wait, I think it might be his undoing. If it takes twenty minutes to ready the plane for takeoff, the airfield is called in advance so that the plane will be all but off the ground the minute he gets there. In the summer, the boat is tugging at anchor. In the winter, every weekend he is on skis from nine in the morning to the last bit of light. The masseur then is at the ready. Now that Marella, his wife, has got him interested in contemporary art, no schedule is too tight to fit in a fast trip to a show.

When you have dinner with the Agnellis, the talk is animated. If you join in at the usual pace, the plates have disappeared before you begin to eat. Gianni eats very little and quickly. He believes in rest, however. When away from the workaday week and off on a cruise, he and Marella sneak off quietly without saying good night when the clock says 10:30 P.M.

At St. Moritz one evening, he remarked, "How strange, I'm extraordinarily tired." I had never heard him say such a thing before. It turned out that he had come down with Asian flu and his temperature was 101 degrees.

His is not a regime to recommend to everyone, but with Gianni it works. Most men have neither the means, the metabolism, nor the desire to go at this pitch. Thank God—I, for one, could never keep up. But I do notice a love of fast pace and self-expenditure in many men who keep their looks; a liking for fine but rather simple food; little or no smoking, not that much drinking, and great importance attached to sex. There are exceptions to all of these rules, and as for making love, in lieu of statistics, I have to conclude that it is the attitude that counts.

Use of makeup is not frequent. Men still prefer sun or sun lamp to produce a glow. Even if they know that too much sun is bad for the skin, they assume theirs can take it better than women's. Regarding men's cosmetics, Max Factor's Gil informed me briskly that men do not make up, they "color" themselves, or at most, they "gloss." The formula he suggests is twice a week under the sun lamp with a protective cream and eye pads with rose water as a base, plus a quick-tan product when you cannot get to the beach or the slopes.

Franco Zeffirelli says that on winter evenings when he feels very tired and has to go out, Braggi's tan gives a lift. Valentino believes in a daily dose of cream and talcum powder. "I was never a boy who hated to be washed behind the ears," he points out. "At sixteen, I started the after-shave routine I use today: After the razor—a real one, not electric—I put Nivea cream on the face and remove it with tissue, then apply talcum powder for fifteen minutes. The skin feels marvelous."

Industrialist Nino Cerruti agrees that putting something good on the face pleases a man just as much as it does a woman. Nino also thinks that a cream to relax the face in the evening would be a good idea for men.

Rudi Crespi defends makeup again, adding that if it seems sissy, one is in such good company. Prominent men who have never lacked for women are now beginning to wear makeup to parties when they are not tanned—even some of the Rothschilds wore it at a masked ball in Paris last year. It is all part of putting back the plumage on males.

And being rather fond of plumage, I asked Carlo Palazzi, Rome's favorite menswear designer, what he thought of the peacock revolution. "We have ruined men a bit. They're wearing too much costume now," he says. "There was a group in the other day and the simplest of the trio had a mink down to his ankles and a diamond chain. You don't have to put curlers in your hair or load yourself down with chains. But the fact is that sticking always to conservative classics is dull and looks wrong."

Palazzi tries to advise men on how far to go. An ex-athlete whose muscles are collapsing should not delude himself that big-shouldered coats and wide pants will disguise the fact. On the other hand, he is not in physical shape for the most fashionable number in a collection and should be dissuaded from buying it. Men often tend to extremes—when they finally decide to stray from classics, they lose all sense of proportion. I wonder how many shirts have had to be accidentally ruined in the wash? How many jackets have you longed to drop acid on?

As anyone in the business has always known, no matter what their taste, men can be just as hysterical about clothes as women. Palazzi thinks this has increased since men have started experimenting with crash diets to lose their girth—and ruined their nerves instead. But there have always been types who take two hours to decide exactly how a seam should be done. (Sometimes a tailor learns a lot from them. Often it is a waste of everyone's time.)

Male narcissism, rarely avowed, has to be taken for granted by a tailor. How else does one explain the customer who has forty fittings for a pair of shorts? The one who has his pajamas custom-made and is never satisfied with them? (Sales of pajamas have been down for years because men do not bother with them anymore.) Or best of all, the client who never tries on anything without stripping to the nude and then putting his shoes back on?

These are fringe cases, perhaps, but I see no

reason why men have to be hypocritical about their vanity. Any woman who has ever lived with a man knows how profound it can be. Male protests to the contrary are such a bore. I think it takes self-assurance, and a good body, to wear some of the best designs and accessories. But plumage never harms the bird. On a real man, it looks great. Exaggerated, on certain homosexuals, it just makes them look more feminine, which was their nature to begin with.

As always, it is a question of type and scale—a peacock is not a pheasant, a flamingo, or a wren. Marcello Mastroianni, who tends to dress quietly and casually in private life, once explained that you do not have to be an actor to wear costume— one of the reasons men used to become actors. But now that everyone can be eccentric and extravagant, he does not want to be.

I do not think it is just to wear clothes well that men make an effort to stay in shape. Nor is it just to have delectable young girls. But I would not say it was just for efficient work performance either. "A healthy mind in a healthy body" does not explain why men sneak in a fast hair comb in public just as women fix up their lipstick. Men's motives are mixed—and long live the results when they are attractive.

Gianni Bulgari, the jeweler, finds it distasteful for men to wear obvious fashion, echoing the ancient fear that it might give the frivolous impression one spends lots of time on it. Probably one spends the same amount of time on looking conservative, but there is no sense arguing with a man who has found a style that becomes him.

Gianni's system for staying in top form is to get

up when he still feels a bit sleepy and to leave the table a bit hungry. He says that this sort of training in little sufferings may seem a bit masochistic, except that you feel worse when you relent. He was a fat teenager, and it still haunts him. Supposedly, the metabolism changes and you are not as hungry in your thirties as in your teens. He suspects that, by nature, he would still be voracious. "Three times a week, I get up at 6:30 to be at the gym by 7:00," he adds. "I will fight a paunch to the last out of self-respect and because a paunch never seduced anyone."

Like many businessmen, he rarely has a month off with nothing to do connected with business. He swims in the summer and used to ski, fence, and box when he had more time. He flies, but his passion now is gliding. There is a center near Rome he drives to on free Sundays. Gliding is not a stay-in-shape duty. It is the most relaxing and challenging sport he knows. "I'd love to go to Texas for a week to glide," he says wistfully. "I never can."

Franco Zeffirelli, who had to curtail swimming and exercise for a period after his accident, confesses that, if he has to go into town to a gym to exercise, he is too lazy. (Franco lives in a rented villa outside Rome and plans to renovate a country house of his own—no more city hassle for him.) He bought a rowing machine, bicycle, weights, and wheels to use at home, but like most people wound up never touching them. The solution is someone who comes to the house; in his case, a tennis coach who lives next door. The coach makes him run in the garden and work up a sweat.

According to Franco, the city you feel best in is New York because you walk there all the time:

"There's always so much to do and you can't stay in an apartment looking at TV." Rudi Crespi, who lives in the center of Rome, finds on the contrary that Villa Borghese is the perfect place to walk for an hour every day. There is no ideal exercise pattern. Whatever fits a man's constitution and schedule and still brings results is the answer. And he has to find it. You cannot tell him.

As Gore Vidal suggests, often the problem is that the way you are built and what you use your body for do not coincide. As a writer, for example, he needs a skinny body and a big head. Instead, he has the Vidal Alpine heritage. The men in the family still have forty-eight-inch chests to pull in oxygen, even if they now live at sea level and all that expansion will be the death of them.

Gore, when in Rome, goes to the gym every afternoon for two hours and has found a masseur who comes to the house several times a week. "After forty, males need gym work for sex purposes," he adds. "After all, sex is largely a matter of circulation." Like most Romans, he likes to devote the evening to conversation, food, and drink. "That American system of cocktail, theater, supper, night-club—and then she surrenders her treasure—leads straight to coronary thrombosis. It is better in the afternoon."

Franco Zeffirelli echoes Gore on the vital importance of sex. He sees it as a great moment of achievement, of human contact, a mutual exchange of energies, an extraordinary chemical experience, the dream, the illusion, the dark room where all men are kings.

At the risk of sounding like a reactionary prude, Franco has blasted pornography and groin films, not because he is against sex for every man, but because he is for it and against total commercialization. "SOS for sex," Franco says. "But it has to remain a private world—what if you no longer cared, no longer looked at someone and wondered what they were like in bed?"

Emilio Pucci puts the case more directly. "Making love is one of the greatest ways of keeping balance," he says. "How many men, stressed and undone by the day, wish they could stop, clap hands, and have sex—no emotional tie, no talking —just sex. How much more amusing it is to go out with a woman who understands without explanations—the kind who can say without any overture on your part, 'No, not here, it's too dangerous.'"

To keep fit, Pucci does not smoke, eats very carefully, and drinks only wine. He thinks a man must keep fit for various reasons. One is that a person of quality simply cannot have a big stomach. Another is that if you work, you are supposed to be all there the moment you get up, which is difficult at any age. Busy men are always under stress more than they can stand. Pucci says he can give up sleep under pressure, but cannot give up feeling—then you are dead.

Sex, no matter how revitalizing, cannot offset stress entirely, and stress takes a toll of anyone's looks. As part of a promotion campaign, a group of beer-drinking centenarians was assembled for a visit to Rome and the Pope some time ago. One of the hundred-year-olds explained their secret: "Even tragedy runs off us like water off marble," he said. "Our emotions no longer work against us."

In this vein, Nino Cerruti finds that the best calmant is simply to look at the sea or the garden—

to be as receptive as possible to the world around us that does not speak. Of course, as a Paris-Milan businessman, he commutes more than communes and therefore also resorts to tranquilizers. With the latter, he finds that sleeping pills are never needed. He sleeps as much as he can (a great beauty treatment, I might add) and firmly believes in the magic properties of everything that happens during sleep.

We all seem to take pills of one kind or another with no harm done as long as they are not abused. Nino takes tranquilizers and scorns vitamins. Franco Zeffirelli, as his English friends well know, is a vitamin fiend. They and anyone else coming to Rome via London are pressed into bringing him supplies of an English brand of vitamin B complex that seems to work best for him. I agree with Franco that vitamins are the healthiest thing to get hooked on. And for anyone exposed to antibiotics or trying to recoup from operations, illness or fatigue, the "B's" are fantastic.

"I'm probably the only man left who doesn't take pep pills, sleeping tablets, tranquilizers, LSD, or marijuana—medicine and drugs, even aspirin, upset my system," he claims. "After four months of antibiotics last year, I was so deprived of defenses, I came down with one infection after another. Vitamin B was my lifeboat. It makes me feel healthy and protects me from my alienations."

As for beauty sleep, Franco says he gets it anywhere, anyhow, and never enough. Like many low-blood-pressure types, he does not get up early if he can avoid it and never falls asleep before two. But when obliged to get up for a good reason, like catching the 7:15 sun for a scene in a film, he adjusts. You have to.

"I have tricks," he explains. "At lunch break, I gnaw quickly on a chicken bone and then sleep for fifty minutes. This gives me a second start. And during the three or four months that shooting lasts, my metabolism changes. Man is a very flexible animal. His life is artificial. He doesn't live in the jungle and wake up like the birds because he feels the dawn."

In addition, both Franco and Nino are simple-food men—most beautiful Italians are. They may eat pasta, but they do not like complicated sauces, international French cuisine, and other pseudo-refinements. Good wines, grilled meat, country soups, and tons of fresh salad and fruits are the staples.

Gore Vidal, living in Rome, has also adopted the simple food habit, particularly for lunch. "Like every American writer I know, I could be an alcoholic," he says. "But I'm not about to destroy myself. For lunch, raw mushrooms and yoghurt are fine. I don't drink, I feel well, and it keeps the weight down."

Rudi Crespi's big discovery of the moment—I do not know how long it will last—is a procaine-based rejuvenation cure. "I feel like I'm twenty-five," he says. "I throw myself in sixty different directions, have all sorts of new interests. What it does for memory is incredible, and the hair that was graying has turned brown again. I even think I'm more intelligent, and Consuelo finds me more elated. Maybe it's just maturity, or being in a good cycle to begin with. Last year when I first tried it, I was so worried about many things, it only made me more nervous and I had to stop."

Rejuvenation cures, cosmetics, fashion, pills, plastic surgery—you name it, it is available for men. Am I in favor? Of course. And a regular regimen, a balance between intake and output, work and repose, clearly is what we all need.

Whatever method they choose, men have to take care of themselves if they are to keep their health and their looks. To do nothing is folly. It is not a question of trying to act at forty like a twenty-year-old, but rather of staying in peak form for one's age.

If looking your best does not necessarily mean you feel better or accomplish more, the contrary also holds true. In the age-old endeavor to keep body and soul together someone has yet to come up with the magic formula. My passion is beauty, and that is what I practice and preach. What really matters is that beauty makes the world a pleasanter place to live in—and people easier to love.

ABOUT THE AUTHOR

LUCIANA PIGNATELLI was born in Rome and educated in Switzerland. She was married to Prince Nicolò Pignatelli Aragona Cortes and is now married to Burt S. Avedon, president of Eve of Roma. She speaks four languages, has been a fashion designer, has two children, and is fashion coordinator for Eve of Roma in Europe. Her picture appears often in the leading fashion magazines.

JEANNE MOLLI, a Philadelphian by birth, is married to the Italian artist, Mario Molli. She is a free-lance journalist with *Newsweek*'s Rome bureau and was formerly on the staff of *The New York Times* and *Ladies' Home Journal*.

WE DELIVER!
And So Do These Bestsellers.